Simple Keto Air Fryer Recipe Collection

Tasty and Inspired Desserts Recipes to Boost your Health

River Hunt

© **Copyright 2020 - All rights reserved.**

The content contained within this book may not be reproduced, duplicated or transmitted without direct written permission from the author or the publisher.

Under no circumstances will any blame or legal responsibility be held against the publisher, or author, for any damages, reparation, or monetary loss due to the information contained within this book. Either directly or indirectly.

Legal Notice:

This book is copyright protected. This book is only for personal use. You cannot amend, distribute, sell, use, quote or paraphrase any part, or the content within this book, without the consent of the author or publisher.

Disclaimer Notice:

Please note the information contained within this document is for educational and entertainment purposes only. All effort has been executed to present accurate, up to date, and reliable, complete information. No warranties of any kind are declared or implied. Readers acknowledge that the author is not engaging in the rendering of legal, financial, medical or professional advice. The content within this book has been derived from various sources. Please consult a licensed professional before attempting any techniques outlined in this book.

By reading this document, the reader agrees that under no circumstances is the author responsible for any losses, direct or indirect, which are incurred as a result of the use of information contained within this document, including, but not limited to, — errors, omissions, or inaccuracies.

Homemade Chelsei Currant Buns..8

Mini Apples and Cranberries Crisp Cakes.................................10

Honey Drizzled Banana Fritters..12

Dessert French Toast with Blackberries....................................14

Peppermint Chocolate Cheesecakes...16

Country Pie with Walnuts..18

Coconut Chips Cookies..20

Baked Fruit compote With Coconut Chips...............................22

Coconut Pancake Cups..24

Pop Tarts with Homemade Strawberry Jam............................26

Old Fashioned Plum Dumplings...28

Coconut Cheesecakes Bites..30

Air Grilled Peaches with Cinnamon sugar Butters..................32

Blueberry Fritters with Cinnamon Sugar..................................34

Cinnamon Streuset Coffeecake...36

Sweet Dought Dippers..38

Classic Brownies Cup Cakes..40

Apricot and Almod Crumble...42

Panettone Pudding Tart..44

Favorite Apple Crisp..46

Chocolate Raspberries Wonton...48

Vanilla Cruberrie muffins..50

Lemon Cup Cakes..52

Egg Custard...54

Vanilla Peanut Butter Cookies	56
Almond Pecan Cookies	58
Choco Almond Cake	60
Walnut Carrot Cake	62
Cream Cheese Cupcakes	64
Tasty Pumpkin Muffins	66
Lemon Blueberry Muffins	68
Choco Butter Brownie	70
Ricotta Cake	72
Cinnamon Nut Muffins	74
Chocolate Cheese Brownie	76
Easy Chocolate Cakes	78
Choco Protein Brownies	80
Sliced Apples	82
Raspberry Cobler	84
Protein Donut Balls	86
Delicious Brownie Cupcakes	88
Blueberry Almond Muffins	90
Almond Lemon Bars	92
Coconut Pumpkin Custard	94
Pumpkin Cookies	96
Vanilla Coconut Cakes	98
Butter Cake	101
Chocolate Brownies	103

Cinnamon Strawberry Muffins..105
Quick Brownies...107

Homemade Chelsea Currant Buns

Cook Time:

50 minutes

Servings: 4

Ingredients:

1/2 pound cake flour

1 teaspoon dry yeast

2 tablespoons granulated sugar

A pinch of sea salt

1/2 cup milk, warm

1 egg, whisked

4 tablespoons butter

1/2 cup dried currants

1 ounce icing sugar

Directions:

1. Mix the flour, yeast, sugar and salt in a bowl; add in milk, egg and 2 tablespoons of butter and mix to combine well.

2. Add lukewarm water as necessary to form a smooth dough. Knead the dough until it is elastic; then, leave it in a warm place to rise for 30 minutes.

3. Roll out your dough and spread the remaining 2 tablespoons of butter onto the dough; scatter dried currants over the dough.

4. Cut into 8 equal slices and roll them up. Brush each bun with a nonstick cooking oil and transfer them to the Air Fryer cooking basket.

5. Cook your buns at 330 degrees F for about 20 minutes, turning them over halfway through the cooking time. Dust with icing sugar before serving.

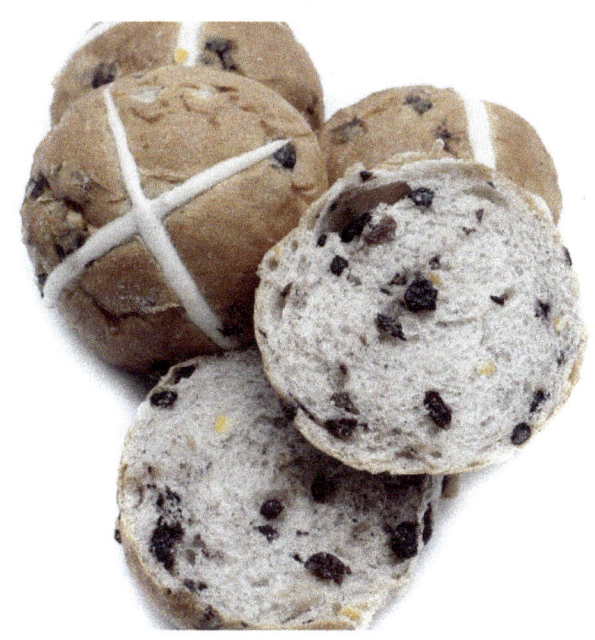

Mini Apple and Cranberry Crisp Cakes

Cook Time:

40 minutes

Servings: 3

Ingredients:

2 Bramley cooking apples, peeled, cored and chopped
1/4 cup dried cranberries

1 teaspoon fresh lemon juice

1 tablespoon golden caster sugar

1 teaspoon apple pie spice mix

A pinch of coarse salt

1/2 cup rolled oats

1/3 cup brown bread crumbs

1/4 cup butter, diced

Directions:

1. Divide the apples and cranberries between three lightly greased ramekins.

2. Drizzle your fruits with lemon juice and sprinkle with caster sugar, spice mix and salt. Then, make the streusel by mixing the remaining ingredients in a bowl.

3. Spread the streusel batter on top of the filling. Bake the mini crisp cakes in the preheated Air Fryer at 330 degrees F for 35 minutes or until they're a dark golden brown around the edges. Enjoy!

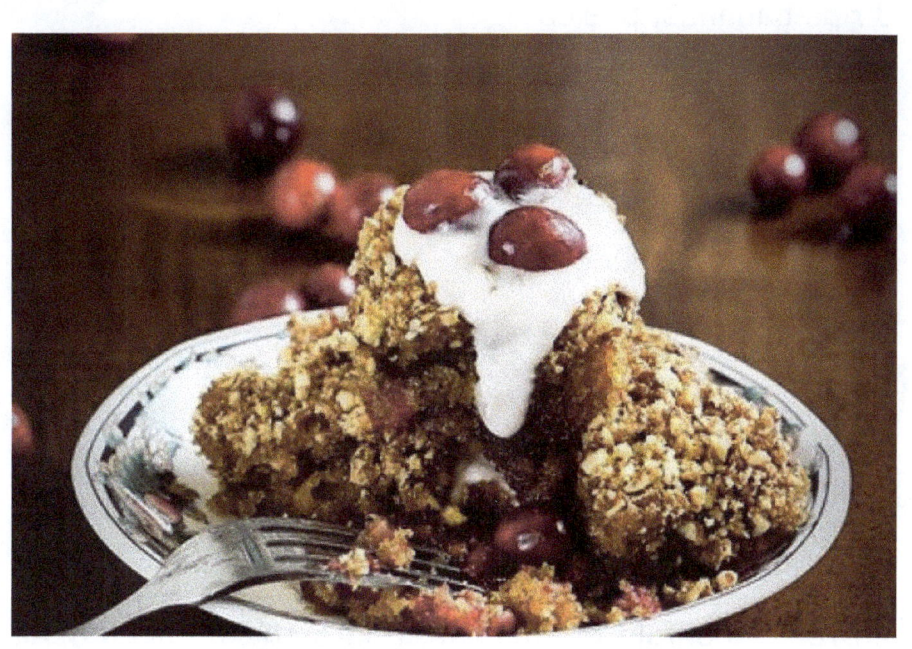

Honey-Drizzled Banana Fritters

Cook Time:

15 minutes

Servings: 3

Ingredients:

3 ripe bananas, peeled

1 egg, whisked

1/4 cup almond flour

1/4 cup plain flour

1/2 teaspoon baking powder

1 teaspoon canola oil

1 tablespoon honey

Directions:

1. Mash your bananas in a bowl. Now, stir in the egg, almond flour, plain flour and baking powder.

2. Drop spoonfuls of the batter into the preheated Air Fryer cooking basket. Brush the fritters with canola oil.

3. Cook the banana fritters at 360 degrees F for 10 minutes, flipping them halfway through the cooking time. Drizzle with some honey just before serving. Enjoy!

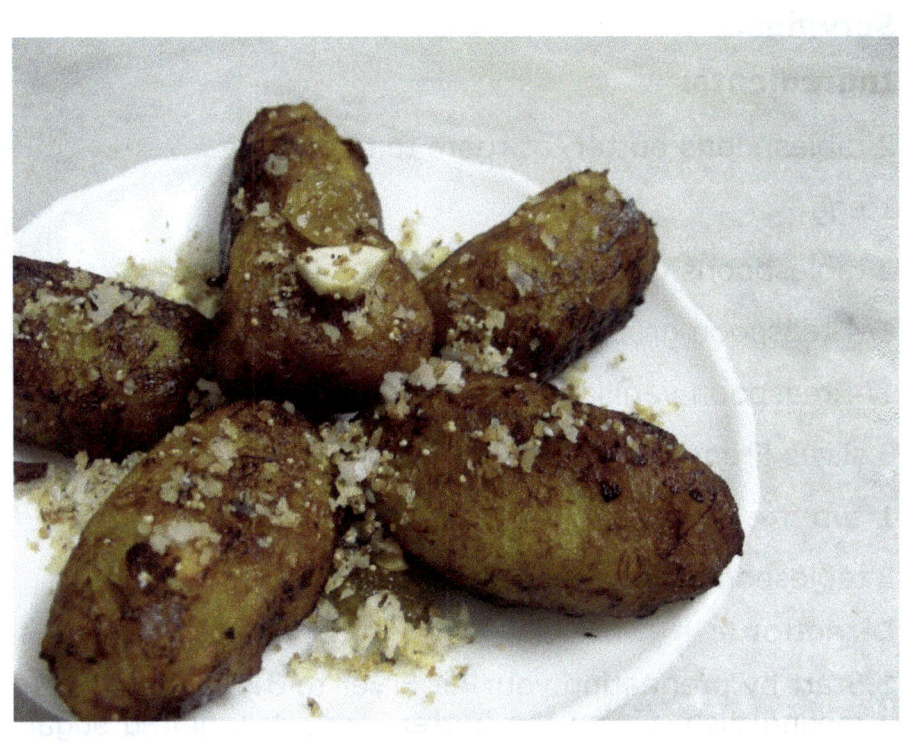

Dessert French Toast with Blackberries

Cook Time:

20 minutes

Servings: 2

Ingredients:

2 tablespoons butter, at room temperature

1 egg

2 tablespoons granulated sugar

1/4 teaspoon ground cinnamon

1/4 teaspoon vanilla extract

6 slices French baguette

1 cup fresh blackberries

2 tablespoons powdered sugar

Directions:

1. Start by preheating your Air Fryer to 375 degrees F. In a mixing dish, whisk the butter, egg, granulated sugar, cinnamon and vanilla.

2. Dip all the slices of the French baguette in this mixture. Transfer the French toast to the baking pan.

3. Bake in the preheated Air Fryer for 8 minutes, turning them over halfway through the cooking time to ensure even cooking.

4. To serve, divide the French toast between two warm plates. Arrange the blackberries on top of each slice. Dust with powdered sugar and serve immediately. Enjoy!

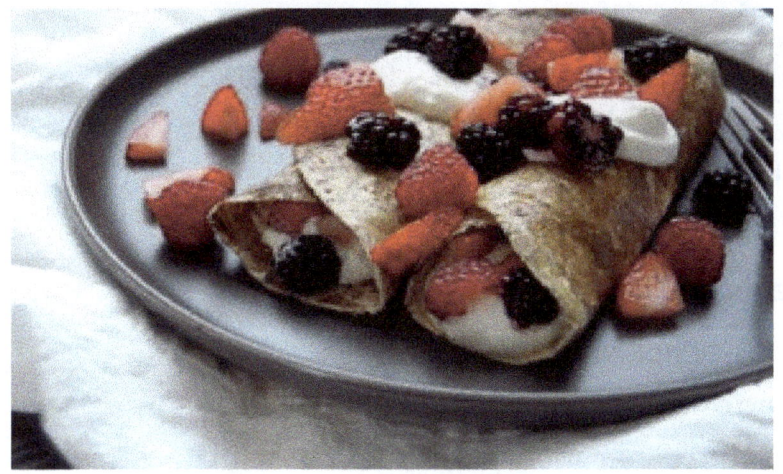

Peppermint Chocolate Cheesecake

Cook Time:

40 minutes

Servings: 6

Ingredients:

1 cup powdered sugar

1/2 cup all-purpose flour

1/2 cup butter

1 cup mascarpone cheese, at room temperature

4 ounces semisweet chocolate, melted

1 teaspoon vanilla extract

2 drops peppermint extract

Directions:

1. Beat the sugar, flour, and butter in a mixing bowl. Press the mixture into the bottom of a lightly greased baking pan.

2. Bake at 350 degrees F for 18 minutes. Place it in your freezer for 20 minutes. Then, make the cheesecake topping by mixing the remaining ingredients.

3. Place this topping over the crust and allow it to cool in your freezer for a further 15 minutes. Serve well chilled.

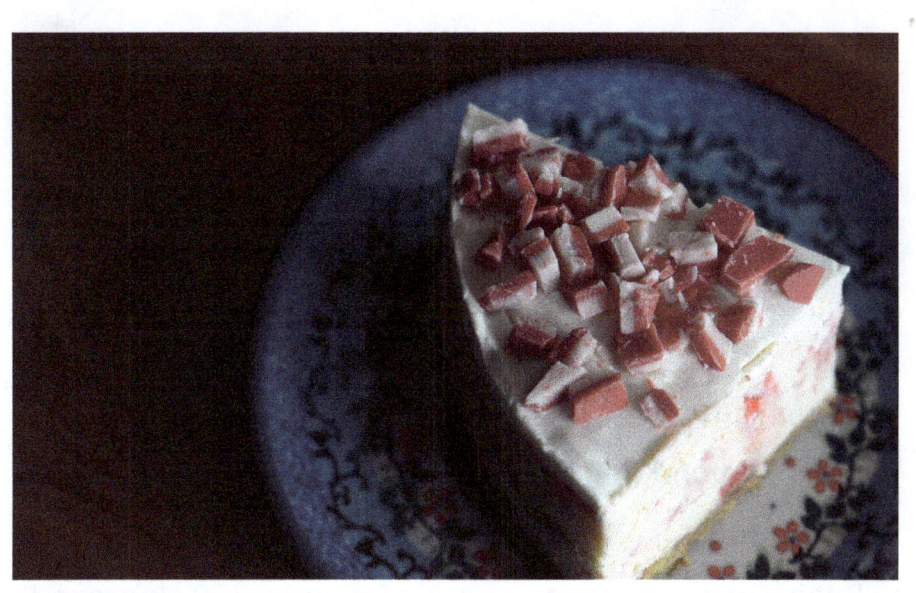

Country Pie with Walnuts

Cook Time:

20 minutes

Servings: 6

Ingredients:

1 cup coconut milk

2 eggs

1/2 stick butter, at room temperature

1 teaspoon vanilla essence

1/4 teaspoon ground cardamom

1/4 teaspoon ground cloves

1/2 cup walnuts, ground

1/2 cup sugar

1/3 cup almond flour

Directions:

1. Begin by preheating your Air Fryer to 360 degrees F. Spritz the sides and bottom of a baking pan with nonstick cooking spray.

2. Mix all ingredients until well combined. Scrape the batter into the prepared baking pan.

3. Bake approximately 13 minutes; use a toothpick to test for doneness. Enjoy!

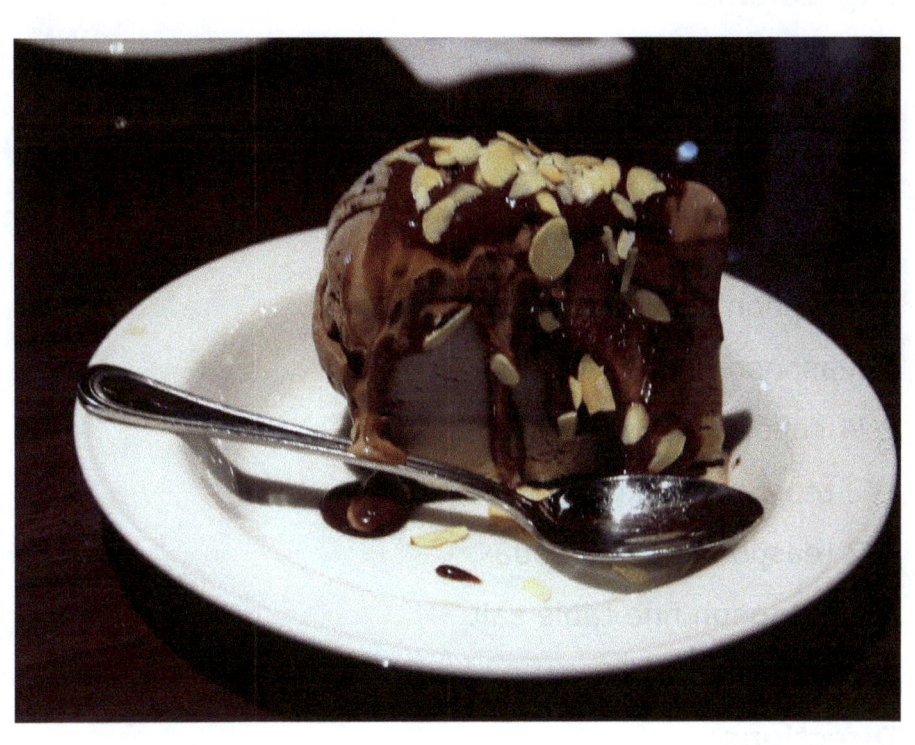

Coconut Chip Cookies

Cook Time:

20minutes

Servings: 12

Ingredients:

1 cup butter, melted

1 ¾ cups granulated sugar

3 eggs

2 tablespoons coconut milk

1 teaspoon coconut extract

1 teaspoon vanilla extract

2 ¼ cups all-purpose flour

1/2 teaspoon baking powder

1/2 teaspoon baking soda

1/2 teaspoon fine table salt

2 cups coconut chips

Directions:

1. Begin by preheating your Air Fryer to 350 degrees F. In the bowl of an electric mixer, beat the butter and sugar until well combined.

2. Now, add the eggs one at a time, and mix well; add the coconut milk, coconut extract, and vanilla; beat until creamy and uniform.

3.Mix the flour with baking powder, baking soda, and salt. Then, stir the flour mixture into the butter mixture and stir until everything is well incorporated.

4.Finally, fold in the coconut chips and mix again. Scoop out 1 tablespoon size balls of the batter on a cookie pan, leaving 2 inches between each cookie.

5.Bake for 10 minutes or until golden brown, rotating the pan once or twice through the cooking time. Let your cookies cool on wire racks. Enjoy!

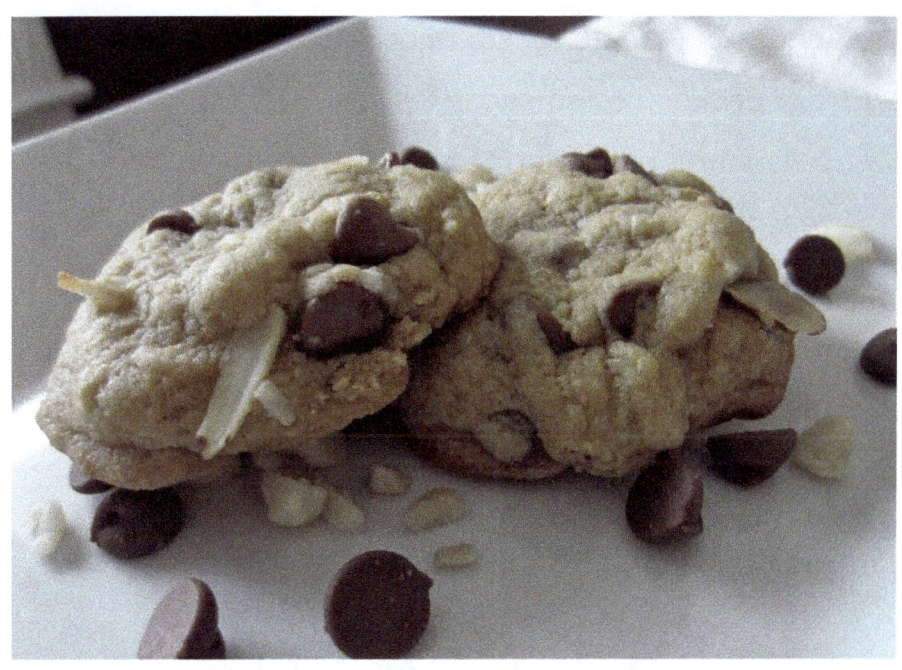

Baked Fruit Compote with Coconut Chips

Cook Time:

25 minutes

Servings: 6

Ingredients:

1 tablespoon butter

8 ounces canned apricot halves, drained

8 ounces canned pear halves, drained

16 ounces pineapple slices, undrained

1/3 cup packed brown sugar

1/4 teaspoon grated nutmeg

1/4 teaspoon ground cloves

1/2 teaspoon ground cinnamon

1 teaspoon pure vanilla extract

1/2 cup coconut chips

Directions:

1. Start by preheating your Air Fryer to 330 degrees F. Grease a baking pan with butter.

2. Place all ingredients, except for the coconut chips, in a baking pan. Bake in the preheated Air Fryer for 20 minutes.

3.Serve in individual bowls, garnished with coconut chips. Enjoy!

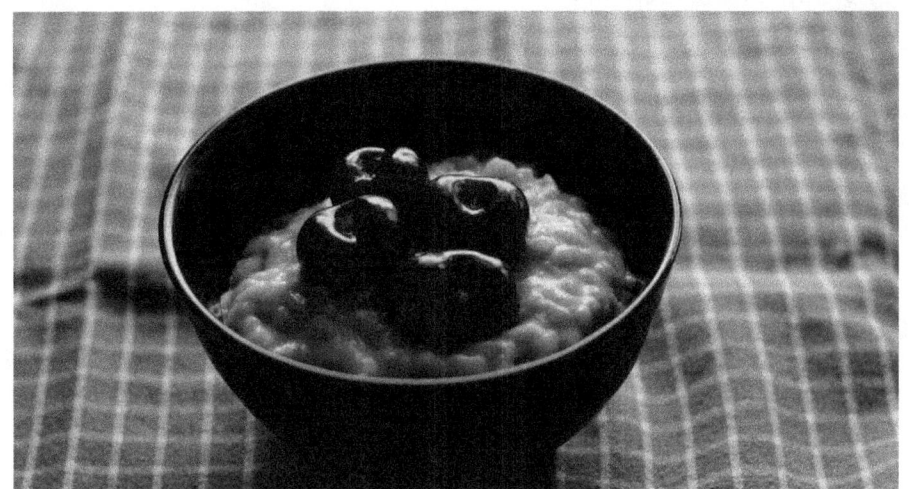

Coconut Pancake Cups

Cook Time:

30 minutes

Servings: 4

Ingredients:

1/2 cup flour

1/3 cup coconut milk

2 eggs

1 tablespoon coconut oil, melted

1 teaspoon vanilla

A pinch of ground cardamom

1/2 cup coconut chips

Directions:

1. Mix the flour, coconut milk, eggs, coconut oil, vanilla, and cardamom in a large bowl.

2. Let it stand for 20 minutes. Spoon the batter into a greased muffin tin.

3. Cook at 230 degrees F for 4 to 5 minutes or until golden brown. Repeat with the remaining batter. Decorate your pancakes with coconut chips. Enjoy!

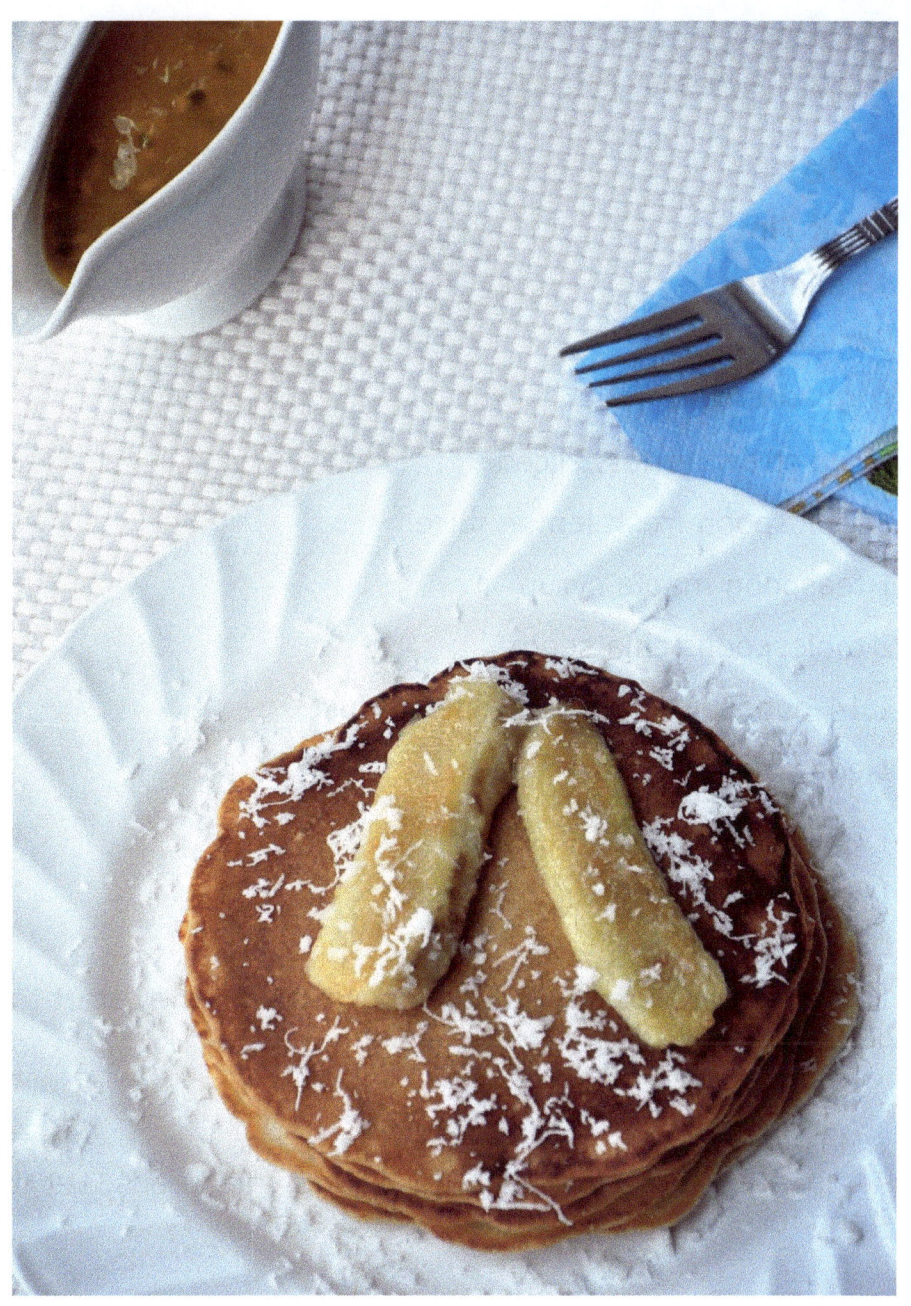

Pop Tarts with Homemade Strawberry Jam

Cook Time:

45 minutes

Servings: 8

Ingredients:

1 cup strawberries, sliced

1 tablespoon fresh lemon juice

1 teaspoon maple syrup

2 tablespoons chia seeds

1 14-ounce box refrigerated pie crust

1 egg, whisked with

1 tablespoon of water egg wash

1/2 cup powdered sugar

Directions:

1. In a saucepan, heat the strawberries until they start to get syrupy.

2. Mash them and add the lemon juice and maple syrup. Remove from the heat and stir in the chia seeds. Let it stand for 30 minutes or until it thickens up.

3. Unroll the pie crusts and cut them into small rectangles. Spoon the strawberry jam in the center of a rectangle; top with another piece of crust.

4.Repeat until you run out of ingredients. Line the Air Fryer basket with parchment paper.

5.Brush the pop tarts with the egg wash and bake at 400 degrees F for 6 minutes or until slightly brown.

6.Work in batches and transfer to cooling racks. Dust with powdered sugar and enjoy!

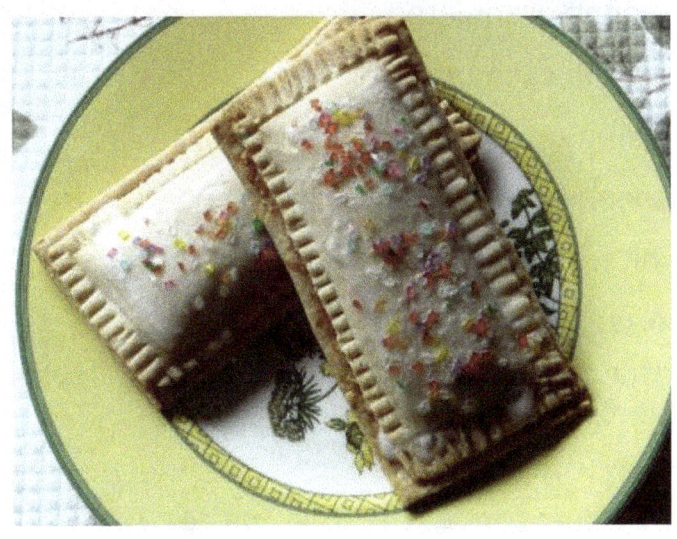

Old-Fashioned Plum Dumplings

Cook Time:

40 minutes

Servings: 4

Ingredients:

1 14-ounce box pie crusts

2 cups plums, pitted

2 tablespoons granulated sugar

2 tablespoons coconut oil

1/4 teaspoon ground cardamom

1/2 teaspoon ground cinnamon

1 egg white, slightly beaten

Directions:

1. Place the pie crust on a work surface. Roll into a circle and cut into quarters.

2. Place 1 plum on each crust piece. Add the sugar, coconut oil, cardamom, and cinnamon. Roll up the sides into a circular shape around the plums.

3. Repeat with the remaining ingredients. Brush the edges with the egg white.

4. Place in the lightly greased Air Fryer basket.

5. Bake in the preheated Air Fryer at 360 degrees F for 20 minutes, flipping them halfway through the cooking time.

6. Work in two batches, decorate and serve at room temperature.

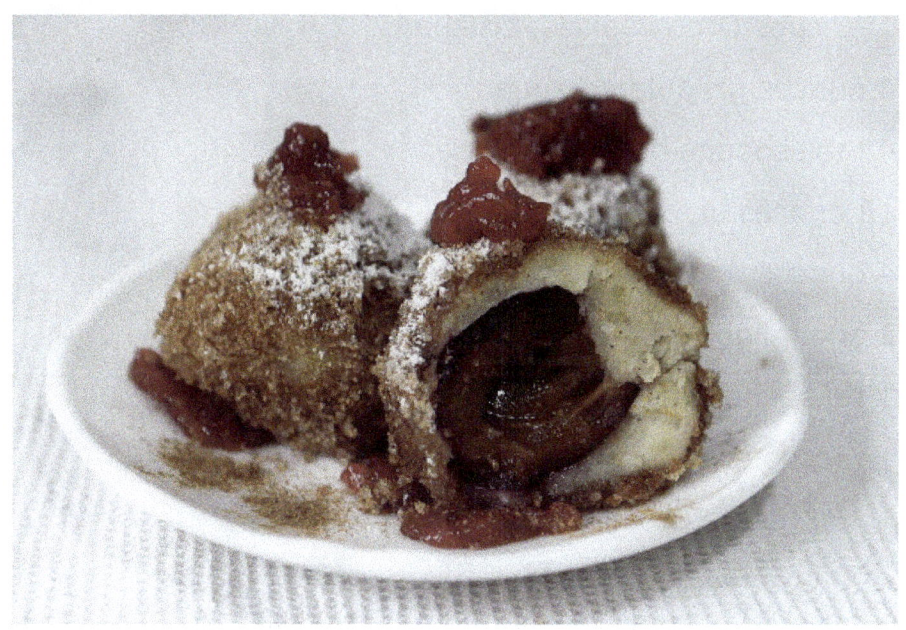

Coconut Cheesecake Bites

Cook Time:

30 minutes

Servings: 8

Ingredients:

1 ½ cups Oreo cookies, crushed

4 ounces granulated sugar

4 tablespoons butter, softened

12 ounces cream cheese

4 ounces double cream

2 eggs, lightly whisked

1 teaspoon pure vanilla extract

1 teaspoon pure coconut extract

1 cup toasted coconut

Directions:

1. Start by preheating your Air Fryer to 350 degrees F. Mix the crushed Oreos with sugar and butter; press the crust into silicone cupcake molds.

2. Bake for 5 minutes and allow them to cool on wire racks. Using an electric mixer, whip the cream cheese and double cream until fluffy; add one egg at a time and continue to beat until creamy.

3. Finally, add the vanilla and coconut extract. Pour the topping mixture on top of the crust. Bake at 320 degrees F for 13 to 15 minutes.

4. Afterwards, top with the toasted coconut. Allow the mini cheesecakes to chill in your refrigerator before serving. Enjoy!

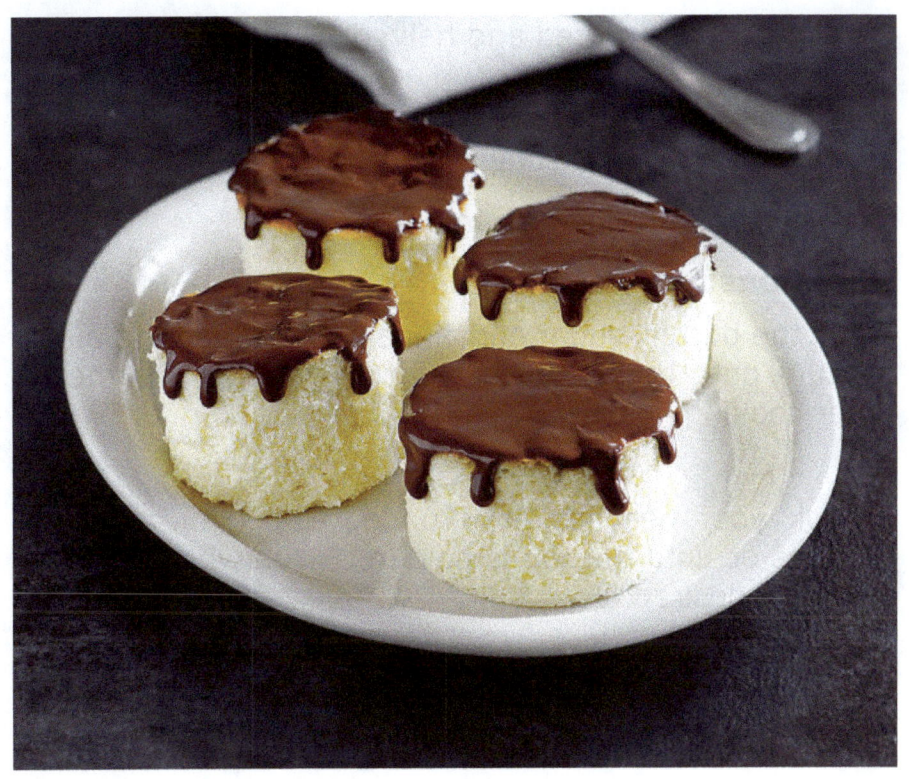

Air Grilled Peaches with Cinnamon-Sugar Butter

Cook Time:

25 minutes

Servings: 2

Ingredients:

2 fresh peaches, pitted and halved

1 tablespoon butter

2 tablespoons caster sugar

1/4 teaspoon ground cinnamon

Directions:

1. Mix the butter, sugar and cinnamon. Spread the butter mixture onto the peaches and transfer them to the Air Fryer cooking basket.

2. Cook your peaches at 320 degrees F for about 25 minutes or until the top is golden. Serve with vanilla ice cream, if desired. Enjoy!

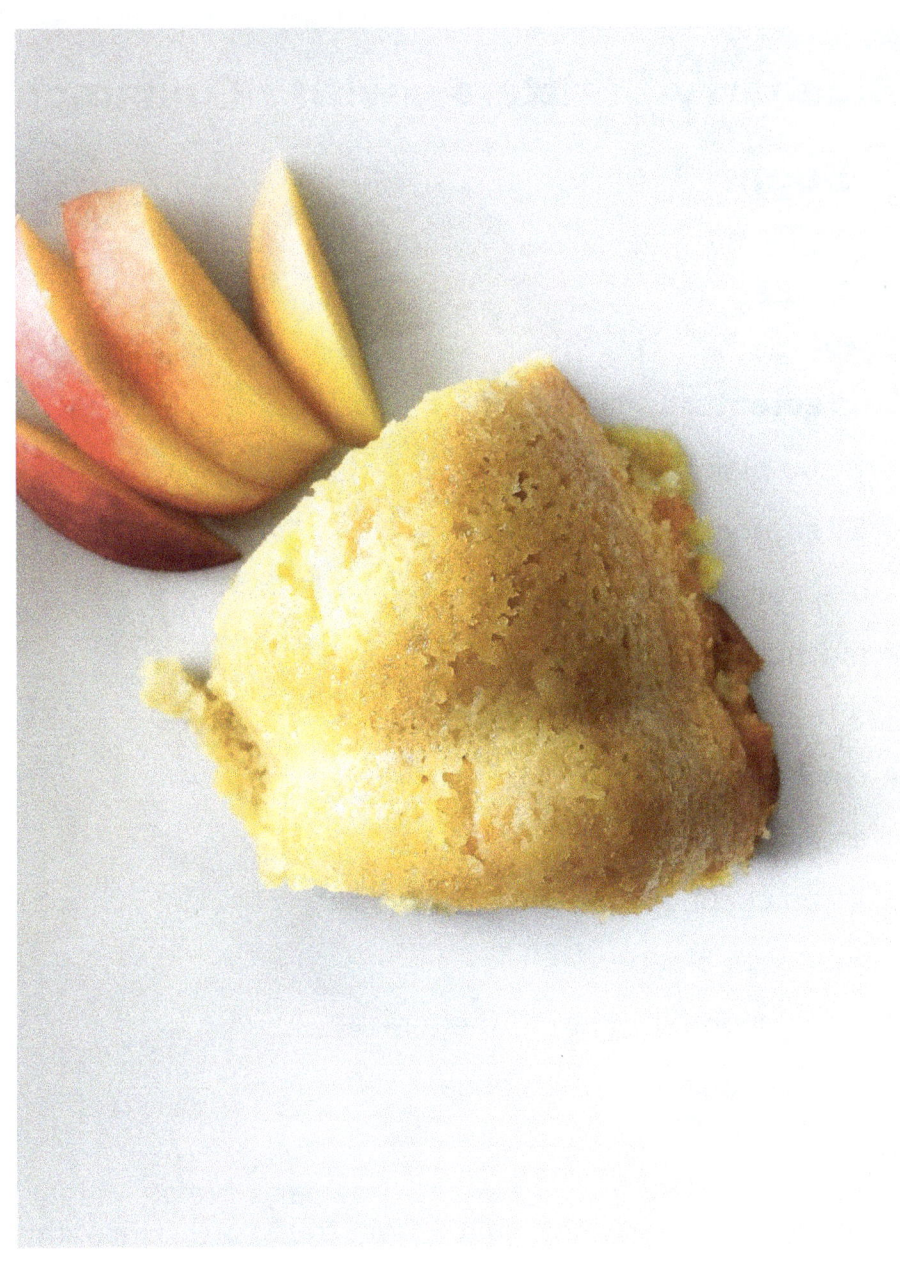

Blueberry Fritters with Cinnamon Sugar

Cook Time:

20minutes

Servings: 4

Ingredients:

1/2 cup plain flour

1/2 teaspoon baking powder

1 teaspoon brown sugar

A pinch of grated nutmeg

1/4 teaspoon ground star anise

A pinch of salt

1 egg

1/4 cup coconut milk

1 cup fresh blueberries

1 tablespoon coconut oil, melted

4 tablespoons cinnamon sugar

Directions:

1.Combine the flour, baking powder, brown sugar, nutmeg, star anise and salt. In another bowl, whisk the eggs and milk until frothy.

2.Add the wet mixture to the dry mixture and mix to combine well. Fold in the fresh blueberries.

3.Carefully place spoonfuls of batter into the Air Fryer cooking basket. Brush them with melted coconut oil.

4.Cook your fritters in the preheated Air Fryer at 370 degrees for 10 minutes, flipping them halfway through the cooking time.

50Repeat with the remaining batter. Dust your fritters with the cinnamon sugar and serve at room temperature. Enjoy!

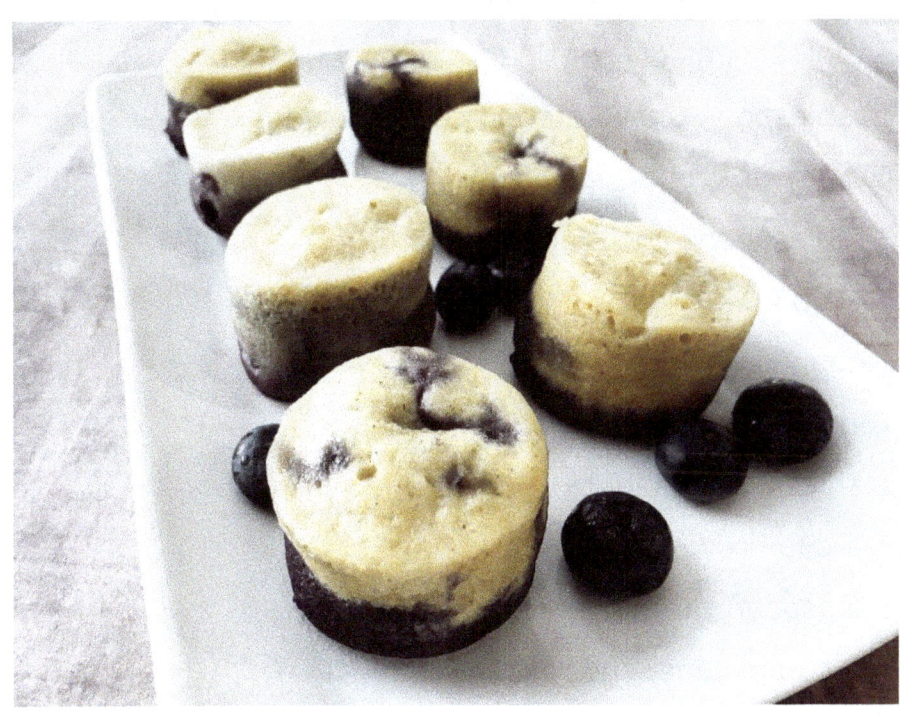

Cinnamon-Streusel Coffeecake

Cook Time:

35 minutes

Servings: 4

Ingredients:

Cake:

1/2 cup unbleached white flour

1/4 cup yellow cornmeal

1 teaspoon baking powder

3 tablespoons white sugar

1 tablespoon unsweetened cocoa powder

A pinch of kosher salt

3 tablespoons coconut oil

14 cup milk

1 egg

Topping:

1tablespoons polenta

1/4 cup brown sugar

1 teaspoon ground cinnamon

1/4 cup pecans, chopped

2 tablespoons coconut oil

Directions:

1. In a large bowl, combine together the cake ingredients. Spoon the mixture into a lightly greased baking pan.

2. Then, in another bowl, combine the topping ingredients. Spread the topping ingredients over your cake.

3. Bake the cake at 330 degrees F for 12 to 15 minutes until a tester comes out dry and clean. Allow your cake to cool for about 15 minutes before cutting and serving. Enjoy!

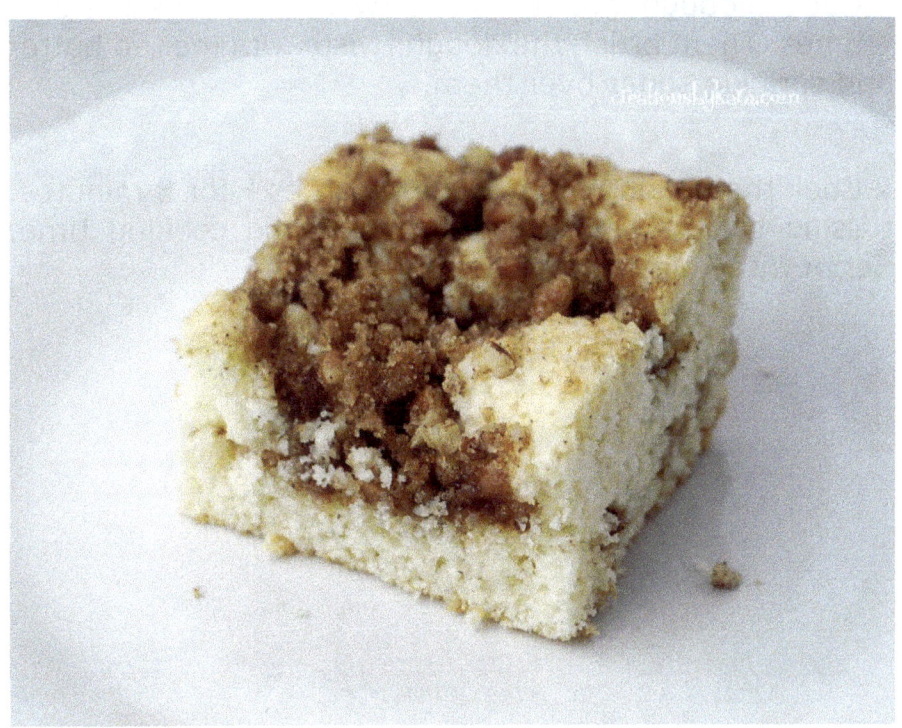

Sweet Dough Dippers

Cook Time:

10 minutes

Servings: 4

Ingredients:

8 ounces bread dough

2 tablespoons butter, melted

2 ounces powdered sugar

Directions

1. Cut the dough into strips and twist them together 3 to 4 times. Then, brush the dough twists with melted butter and sprinkle sugar over them.

2. Cook the dough twists at 350 degrees F for 8 minutes, tossing the basket halfway through the cooking time. Serve with your favorite dip. Enjoy!

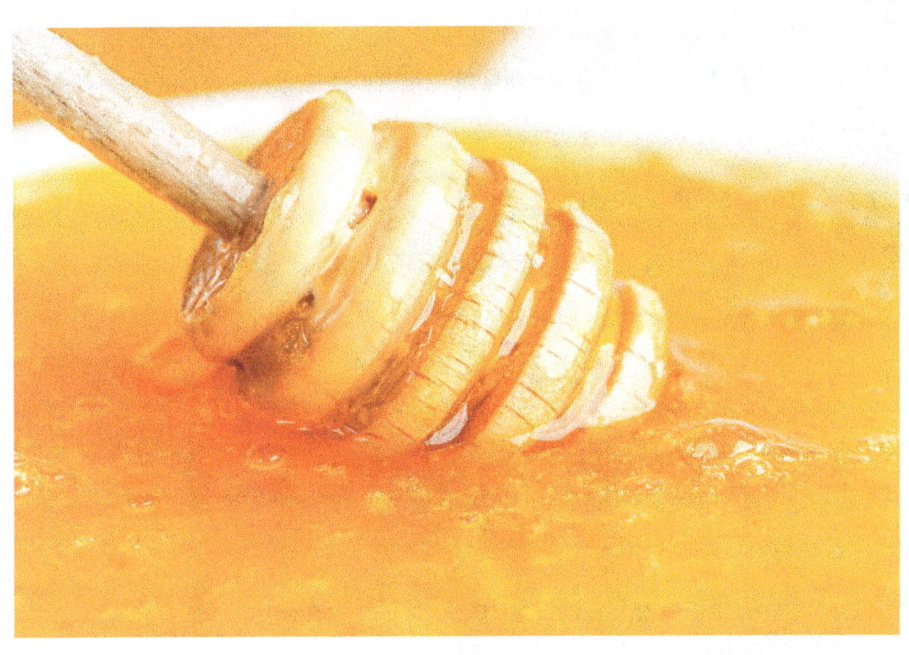

Classic Brownie Cupcakes

Cook Time:

25 minutes

Servings: 3

Ingredients:

1/3 cup all-purpose flour

1/4 teaspoon baking powder

3 tablespoons cocoa powder

1/3 cup caster sugar

2 ounces butter, room temperature

1 large egg

1/2 teaspoon rum extract

A pinch of ground cinnamon

A pinch of salt

Directions:

1. Mix the dry ingredients in a bowl. In another bowl, mix the wet ingredients. Gradually, stir in the wet ingredients into the dry mixture.

2. Divide the batter among muffin cups and transfer them to the Air Fryer cooking basket.

3. Bake your cupcakes at 330 degrees for 15 minuets until a tester comes out dry and clean. Transfer to a wire rack and let your cupcakes sit for 10 minutes before unmolding. Enjoy!

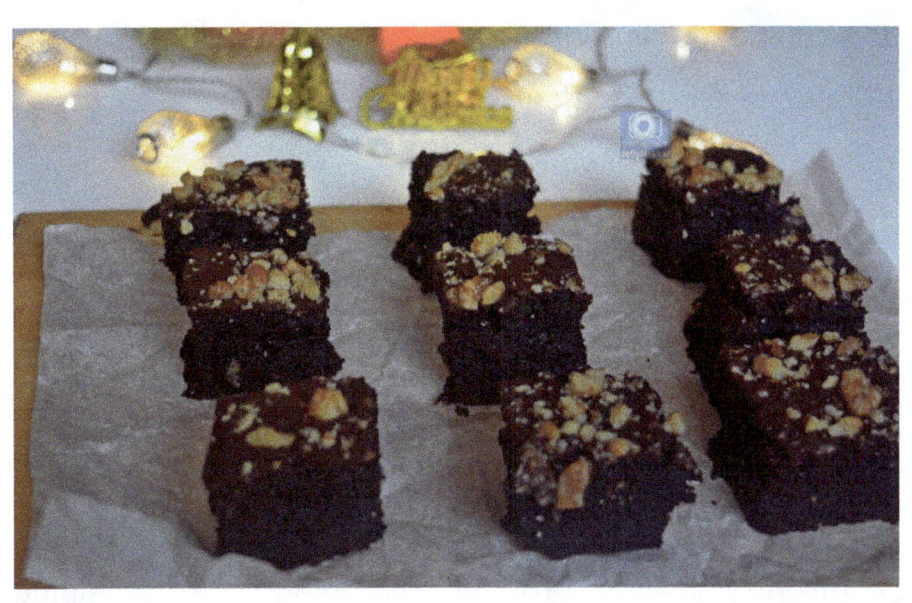

Apricot and Almond Crumble

Cook Time:

35 minutes

Servings: 3

Ingredients:

1 cup apricots, pitted and diced

1/4 cup flaked almonds

1/3 cup self-raising flour

4 tablespoons granulated sugar

1/2 teaspoon ground cinnamon

1 teaspoon crystallized ginger

1/2 teaspoon ground cardamom

2 tablespoons butter

Directions:

1. Place the sliced apricots and almonds in a baking pan that is lightly greased with a nonstick cooking spray. In a mixing bowl, thoroughly combine the remaining ingredients.

2. Sprinkle this topping over the apricot layer. Bake your crumble in the preheated Air Fryer at 330 degrees F for 35 minutes. Enjoy!

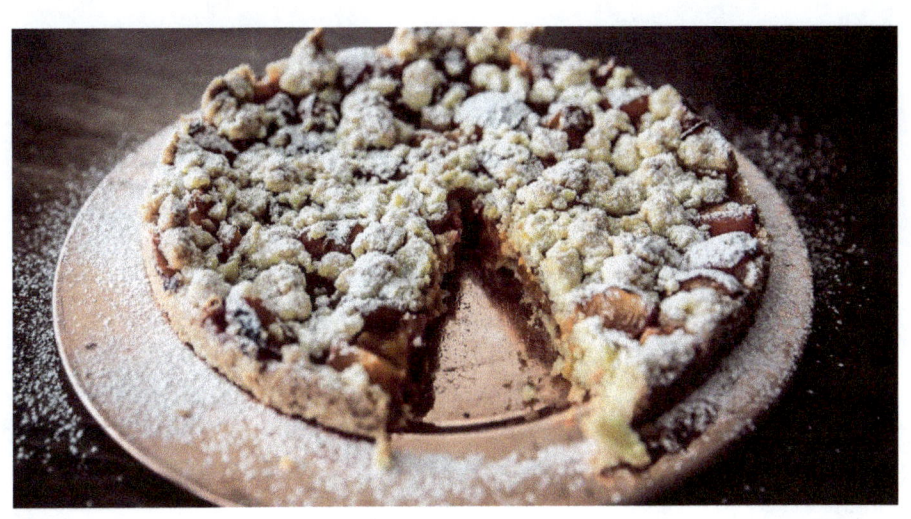

Panettone Pudding Tart

Cook Time:

45minutes

Servings: 3

Ingredients:

3 cups panettone bread, crusts trimmed, bread cut into 1-inch cubes

1/2 cup creme fraiche

1/2 cup coconut milk

2 tablespoons orange marmalade

1 tablespoon butter

2 tablespoons amaretto liqueur

1/2 teaspoon vanilla extract

1/4 cup sugar

A pinch of grated nutmeg

A pinch of sea salt

1 egg, whisked

Directions:

1. Put the panettone bread cubes into a lightly greased baking pan.

2. Then, make the custard by mixing the remaining ingredients. Pour the custard over your panettone.

3.Let it rest for 30 minutes, pressing with a wide spatula to submerge.

4.Cook the panettone pudding in the preheated Air Fryer at 370 degrees F degrees for 7 minutes; rotate the pan and cook an additional 5 to 6 minutes. Enjoy!

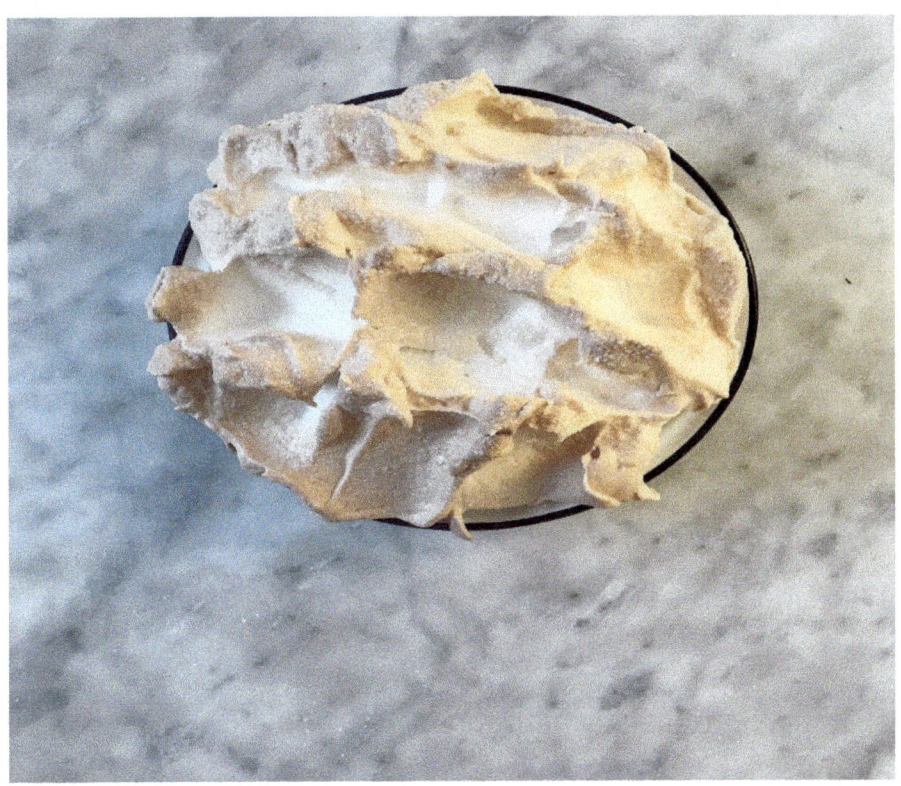

Favorite Apple Crisp

Cook Time:

40minutes

Servings: 4

Ingredients:

4 cups apples, peeled, cored and sliced

1/2 cup brown sugar

1 tablespoon honey

1 tablespoon cornmeal

1/4 teaspoon ground cloves

1/2 teaspoon ground cinnamon

1/4 cup water

1/2 cup quick-cooking oats

1/2 cup all-purpose flour

1/2 cup caster sugar

1/2 teaspoon baking powder

1/3 cup coconut oil, melted

Directions:

1.Toss the sliced apples with the brown sugar, honey, cornmeal, cloves, and cinnamon.

2.Divide between four custard cups coated with cooking spray. In a mixing dish, thoroughly combine the remaining ingredients.

3.Sprinkle over the apple mixture. Bake in the preheated Air Fryer at 330 degrees F for 35 minutes. Enjoy!

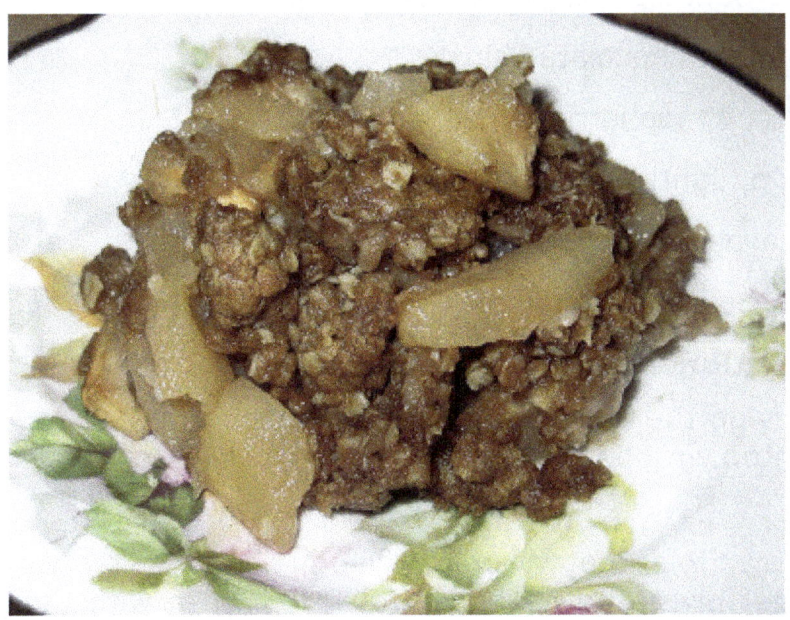

Chocolate Raspberry Wontons

Cook Time:

15minutes

Servings:6

Ingredients:

1 12-ounce package wonton wrappers

6 ounces chocolate chips

1/2 cup raspberries, mashed

1 egg, lightly whisked + 1 tablespoon of water

egg wash

1/4 cup caster sugar

Directions:

1.Divide the chocolate chips and raspberries among the wonton wrappers.

2.Now, fold the wrappers diagonally in half over the filling; press the edges with a fork. Brush with the egg wash and seal the edges.

3.Bake at 370 degrees F for 8 minutes, flipping them halfway through the cooking time. Work in batches. Sprinkle the caster sugar over your wontons and enjoy!

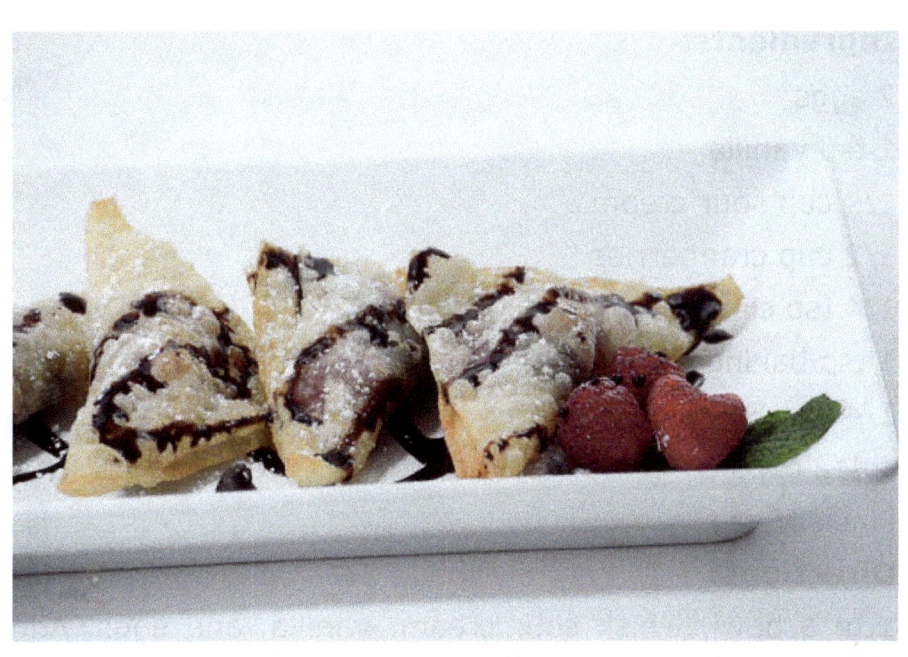

Vanilla Cranberry Muffins

Preparation Time:

10 minutes

Cooking Time:

30 minutes

Serve: 6

Ingredients:

2 eggs

1 tsp vanilla

1/4 cup sour cream

1/2 cup cranberries

1/4 tsp cinnamon

1 tsp baking powder

1/4 cup Swerve

1 1/2 cups almond flour

Pinch of salt

Directions:

1. In a bowl, whisk sour cream, vanilla, and eggs. Add remaining ingredients except for cranberries and beat until smooth.

2. Add cranberries and fold well. Pour batter into the silicone muffin molds. Select Bake mode. Set time to 30 minutes and temperature 325 F then press START.

3.The air fryer display will prompt you to ADD FOOD once the temperature is reached then place muffin molds in the air fryer basket. Serve and enjoy.

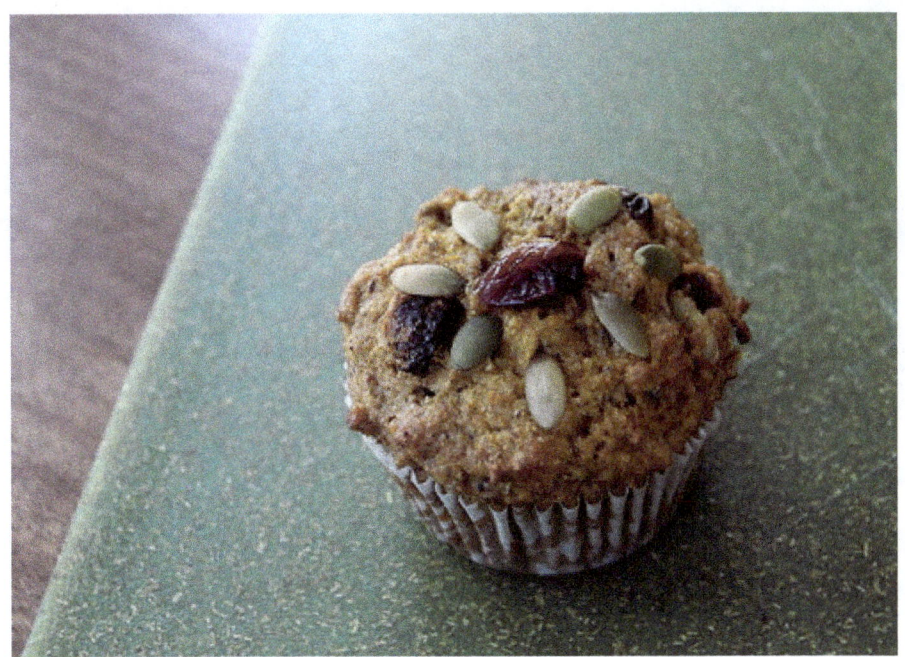

Lemon Cupcakes

Preparation Time:

10 minutes

Cooking Time:

15 minutes

Serve: 12

Ingredients:

2 eggs

1 cup almond flour

1/3 cup Erythritol

1 fresh lemon juice

1 tbsp lemon zest

1/3 cup butter, melted

1/2 cup yogurt

2 tbsp poppy seeds

1 tsp baking powder

1/4 cup coconut flour

Directions:

1. Add all ingredients into the mixing bowl and mix until well combined.

2. Pour batter into the silicone muffin molds. Select Bake mode. Set time to 15 minutes and temperature 350 F then press START.

3.The air fryer display will prompt you to ADD FOOD once the temperature is reached then place muffin molds in the air fryer basket. Serve and enjoy.

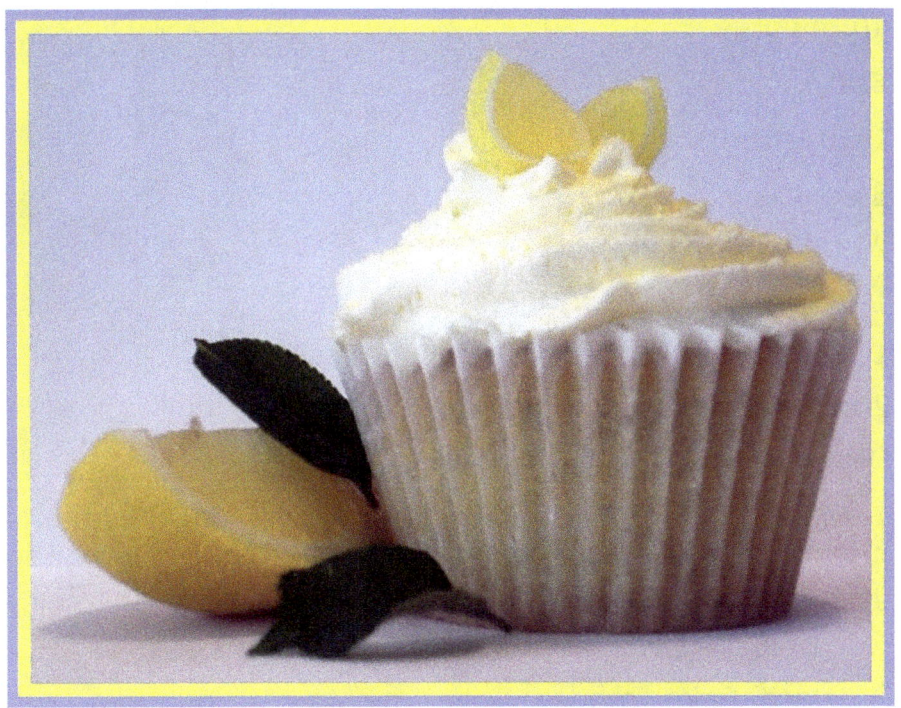

Egg Custard

Preparation Time:

10 minutes

Cooking Time:

40 minutes

Serve: 6

Ingredients:

3 eggs

2 egg yolks

1 tsp vanilla

1/2 cup Swerve

2 cups heavy whipping cream

Directions:

1. Add all ingredients into the large bowl and beat until just well combined. Pour custard mixture into the greased pie dish.

2. Select Bake mode. Set time to 40 minutes and temperature 350 F then press START.

3. The air fryer display will prompt you to ADD FOOD once the temperature is reached then place the pie dish in the air fryer basket. Place custard in the refrigerator for 2 hours. Slice and serve.

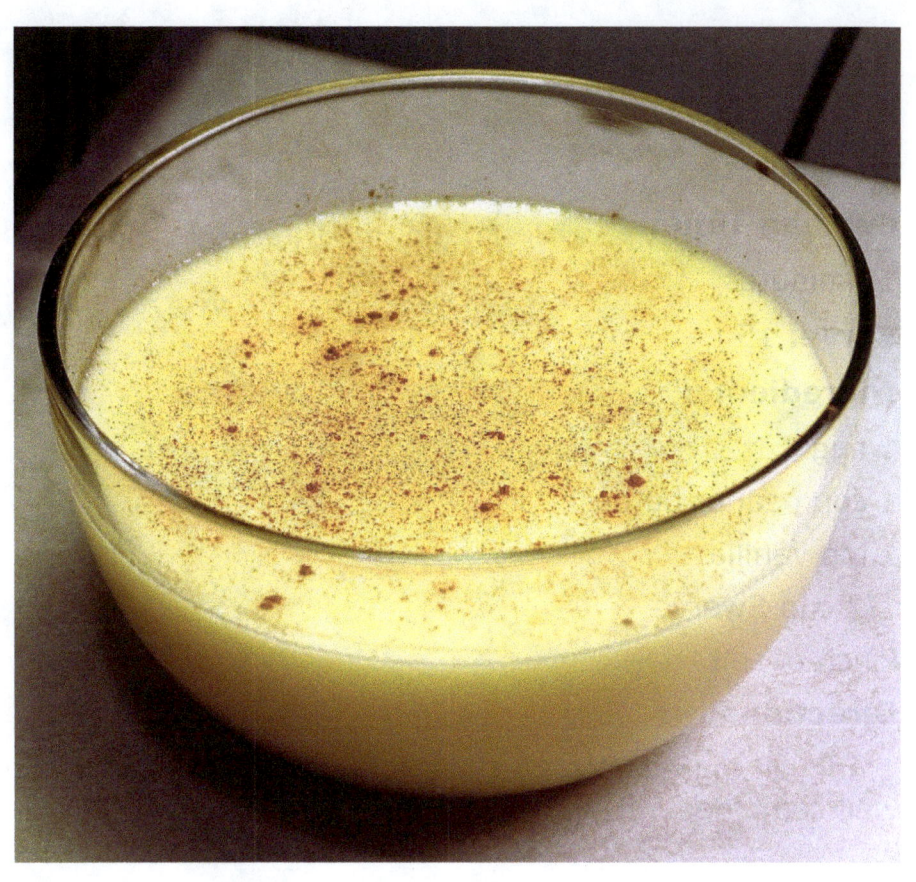

Vanilla Peanut Butter Cookies

Preparation Time:

10 minutes

Cooking Time:

12 minutes

Serve: 15

Ingredients:

1 egg

1 cup peanut butter

1 tsp vanilla

1/2 cup Swerve

Pinch of salt

Directions:

1. Add all ingredients into the large bowl and mix until well combined.

2. Make cookies from the mixture. Place the cooking tray in the air fryer basket. Line air fryer basket with parchment paper.

3. Select Bake mode. Set time to 12 minutes and temperature 350 F then press START.

4. The air fryer display will prompt you to ADD FOOD once the temperature is reached then place cookies onto the parchment paper in the air fryer basket. Serve and enjoy.

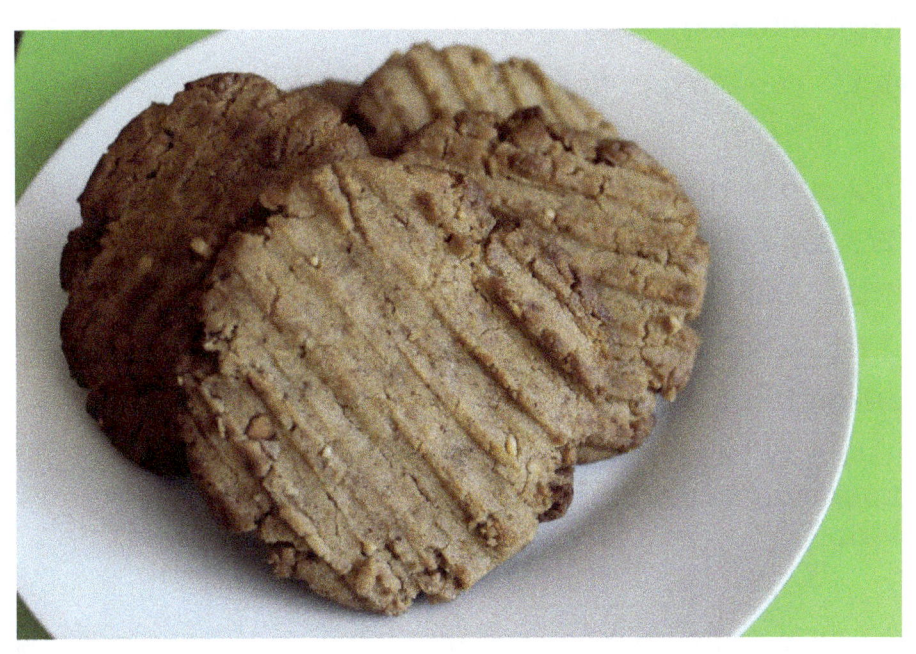

Almond Pecan Cookies

Preparation Time:

10 minutes

Cooking Time:

20 minutes

Serve: 16

Ingredients:

1 1/3 cup almond flour

1 cup pecans

1/2 cup butter

2/3 cup erythritol

1 tsp vanilla

2 tsp gelatin

Directions:

1. Add butter, vanilla, gelatin, sweetener, and almond flour into the food processor and process until crumbs form.

2. Add pecans and process until chopped. Make cookies from the mixture. Place the cooking tray in the air fryer basket.

3. Line air fryer basket with parchment paper. Select Bake mode. Set time to 20 minutes and temperature 350 F then press START.

4. The air fryer display will prompt you to ADD FOOD once the temperature is reached then place cookies onto the parchment paper in the air fryer basket. Serve and enjoy

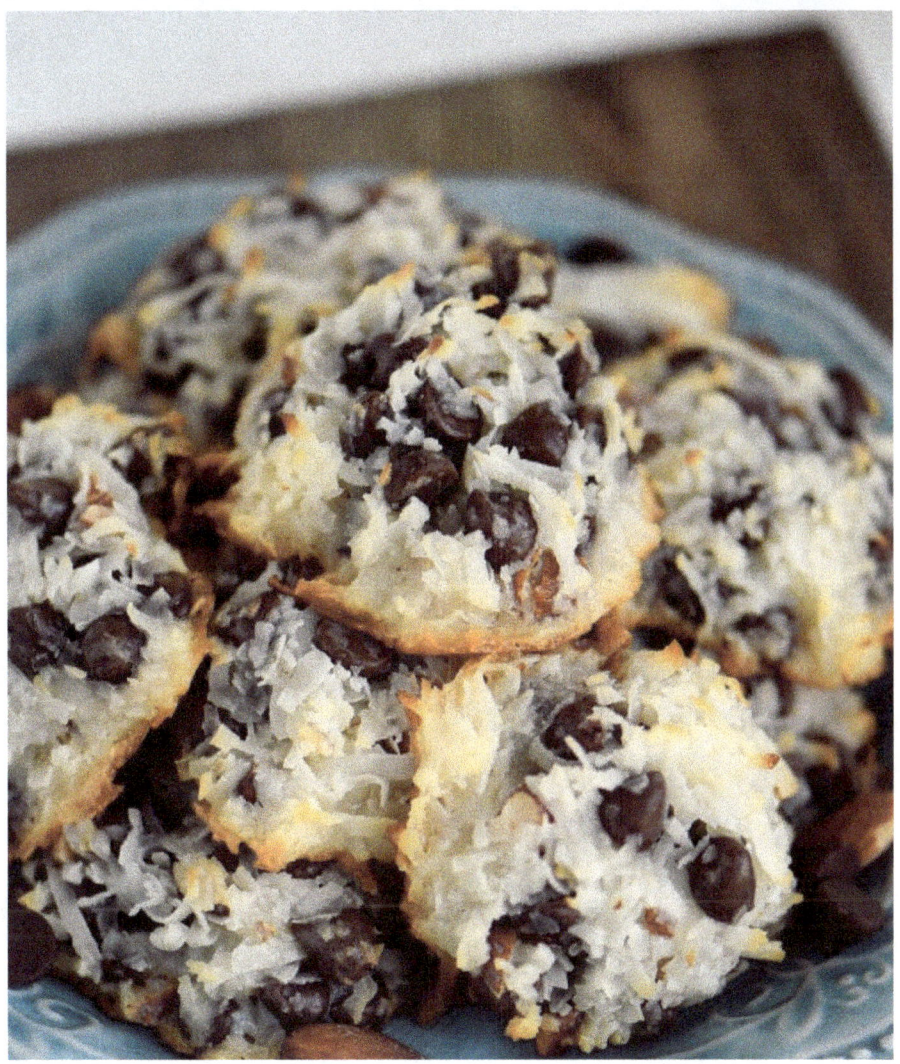

Choco Almond Cake

Preparation Time:

10 minutes

Cooking Time:

20 minutes

Serve: 8

Ingredients:

2 eggs

1/2 cup almond flour

1/2 cup butter, melted

1 tsp vanilla

1/4 cup unsweetened cocoa powder

3/4 cup Erythritol Pinch of salt

Directions:

1. In a bowl, mix together almond flour, cocoa powder, and salt.

2. In a separate bowl, whisk eggs, vanilla extract, and sweetener until creamy.

3. Slowly fold the almond flour mixture into the egg mixture and stir to combine.

4. Add melted butter and stir well. Pour batter into the greased 8-inch baking dish. Select Bake mode.

5.Set time to 20 minutes and temperature 350 F then press START.

6.The air fryer display will prompt you to ADD FOOD once the temperature is reached then place the baking dish in the air fryer basket. Slice and serve.

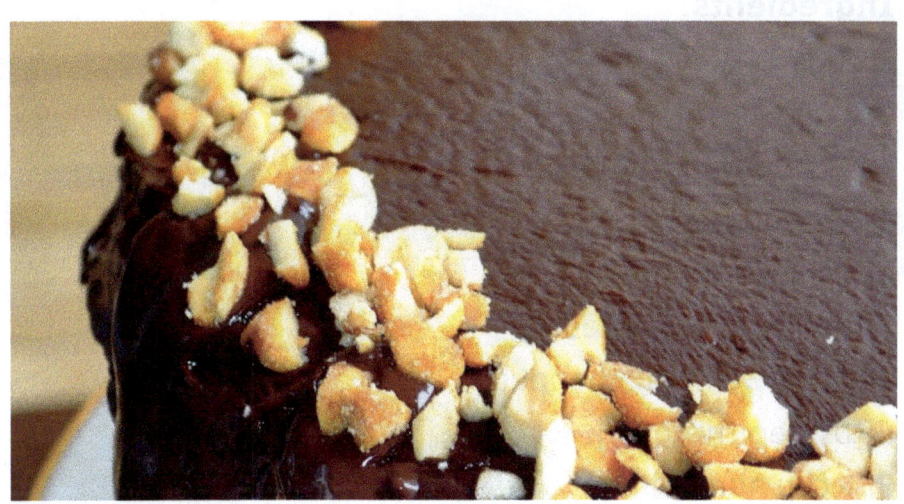

Walnut Carrot Cake

Preparation Time:

10 minutes

Cooking Time:

35 minutes

Serve: 16

Ingredients:

2 eggs

1/2 cup carrots, grated

1/8 tsp ground cloves

1 tsp cinnamon

1 tsp baking powder

2 tbsp butter, melted

1/4 cup walnuts, chopped

6 tbsp erythritol

3/4 cup almond flour

2 tbsp unsweetened shredded coconut

1/2 tsp vanilla Pinch of salt

Directions:

1.In a large bowl, mix together almond flour, cloves, cinnamon, baking powder, shredded coconut, nuts, sweetener, and salt.

2.Stir in eggs, vanilla, butter, and shredded coconut until well combined.

3.Pour batter into the greased baking dish. Select Bake mode. Set time to 35 minutes and temperature 325 F then press START.

4.The air fryer display will prompt you to ADD FOOD once the temperature is reached then place the baking dish in the air fryer basket. Slice and serve.

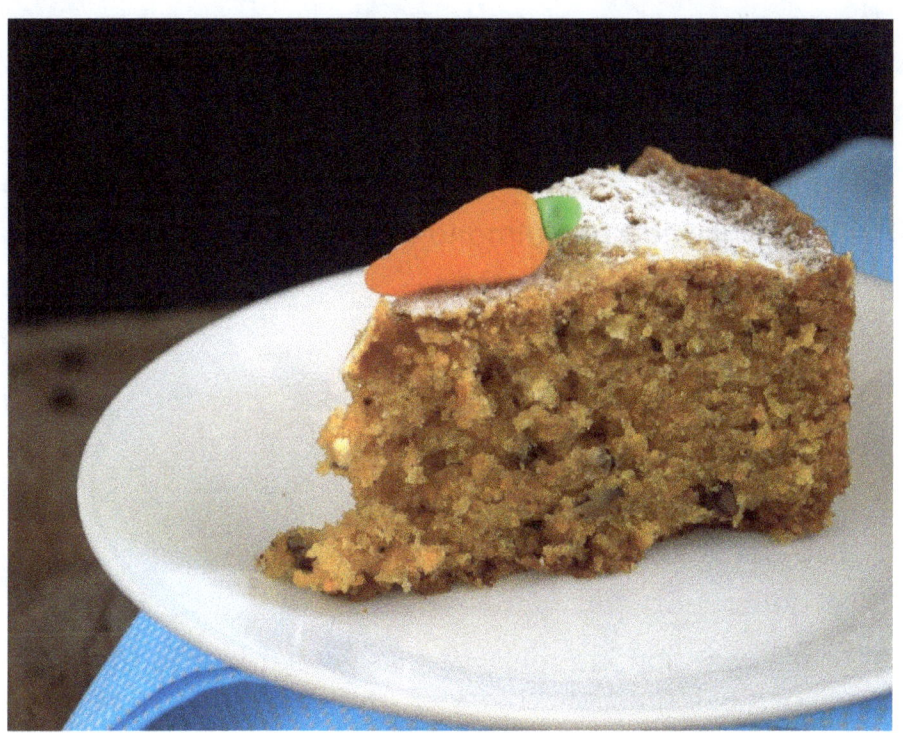

Walnut Muffins

Preparation Time:

10 minutes

Cooking Time:

15 minutes

Serve: 12

Ingredients:

4 eggs

1/2 cup walnuts, chopped

1 1/2 cups almond flour

1 tsp vanilla

1/4 cup unsweetened almond milk

2 tbsp butter, melted

1/2 cup Swerve

1 tsp psyllium husk

1/2 tsp ground cinnamon

2 tsp allspice

1 tbsp baking powder

Directions:

1. Beat eggs, almond milk, vanilla, sweetener, and butter in a bowl using a hand blender until smooth.

2. Add remaining ingredients and stir until well combined. Pour batter into silicone muffin molds.

3. Select Bake mode. Set time to 15 minutes and temperature 400 F then press START.

4. The air fryer display will prompt you to ADD FOOD once the temperature is reached then place muffin molds in the air fryer basket. Serve and enjoy.

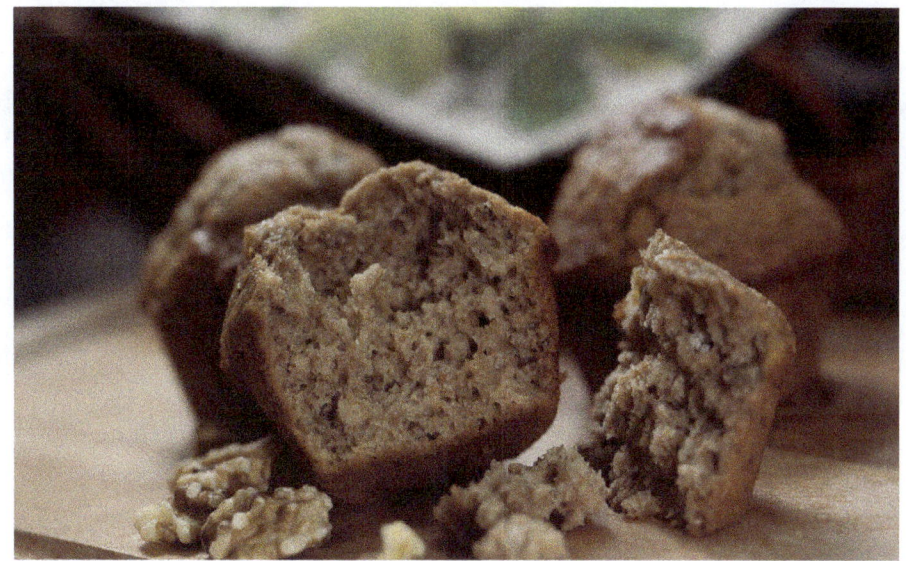

Cream Cheese Cupcakes

Preparation Time:

10 minutes

Cooking Time:

20 minutes

Serve: 10

Ingredients:

2 eggs

8 oz cream cheese

1/2 tsp vanilla extract

1/2 cup Swerve

Directions:

1. In a bowl, mix together cream cheese, vanilla, Swerve, and eggs until soft.

2. Pour batter into the silicone muffin molds Select Air Fry mode. Set time to 20 minutes and temperature 350 F then press START.

3. The air fryer display will prompt you to ADD FOOD once the temperature is reached then place muffin molds in the air fryer basket. Serve and enjoy.

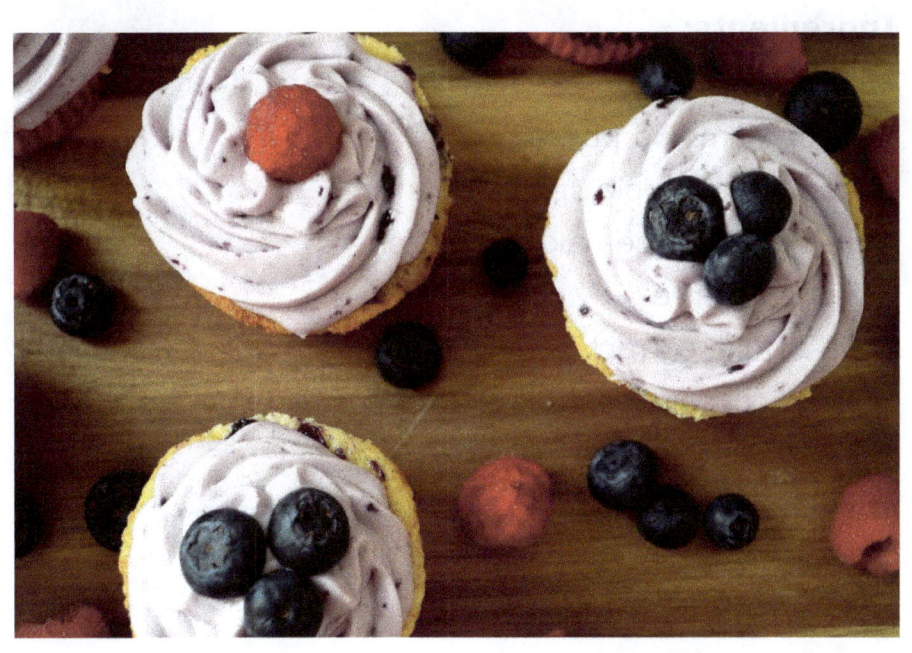

Tasty Pumpkin Muffins

Preparation Time:

10 minutes

Cooking Time:

25 minutes

Serve: 10

Ingredients:

4 large eggs

1/2 cup pumpkin puree

1 tbsp pumpkin pie spice

1 tbsp gluten-free baking powder

2/3 cup Swerve

1 tsp vanilla extract

1/3 cup coconut oil, melted

1/2 cup almond flour

1/2 cup coconut flour

1/2 tsp sea salt

Directions:

1.In a large bowl, stir together coconut flour, pumpkin pie spice, baking powder, erythritol, almond flour, and sea salt.

2.Stir in eggs, vanilla, coconut oil, and pumpkin puree until well combined. Pour batter into the silicone muffin molds.

3.Select Bake mode. Set time to 25 minutes and temperature 350 F then press START.

4.The air fryer display will prompt you to ADD FOOD once the temperature is reached then place muffin molds in the air fryer basket. Serve and enjoy.

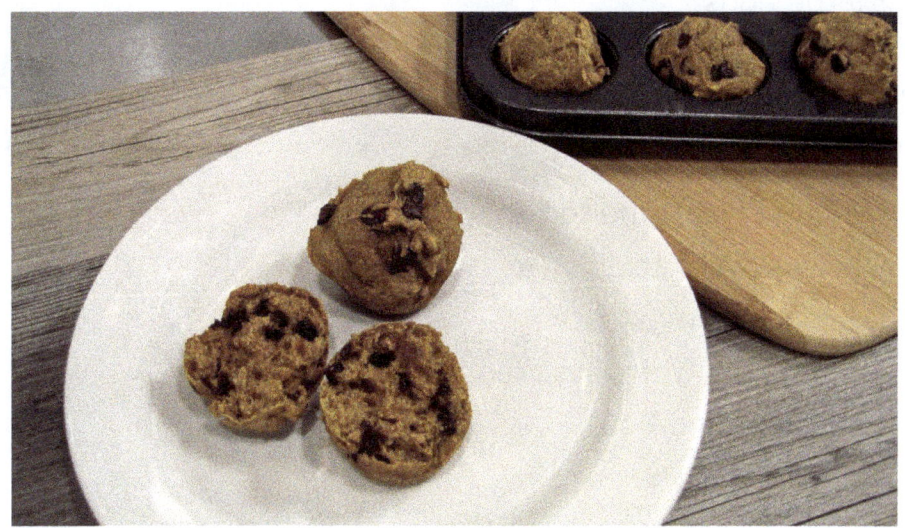

Lemon Blueberry Muffins

Preparation Time:

10 minutes

Cooking Time:

25 minutes

Serve: 12

Ingredients:

2 large eggs

1/2 cup fresh blueberries

1 tsp baking powder

5 drops stevia

1/4 cup butter, melted

1/4 tsp lemon zest

1/2 tsp lemon extract

1 cup heavy whipping cream

2 cups almond flour

Directions:

1. Add eggs to the mixing bowl and whisk until good mix. Add remaining ingredients to the eggs and mix well to combine.

2. Pour batter into the silicone muffin molds. Select Bake mode. Set time to 25 minutes and temperature 350 F then press START.

3. The air fryer display will prompt you to ADD FOOD once the temperature is reached then place muffin molds in the air fryer basket. Serve and enjoy.

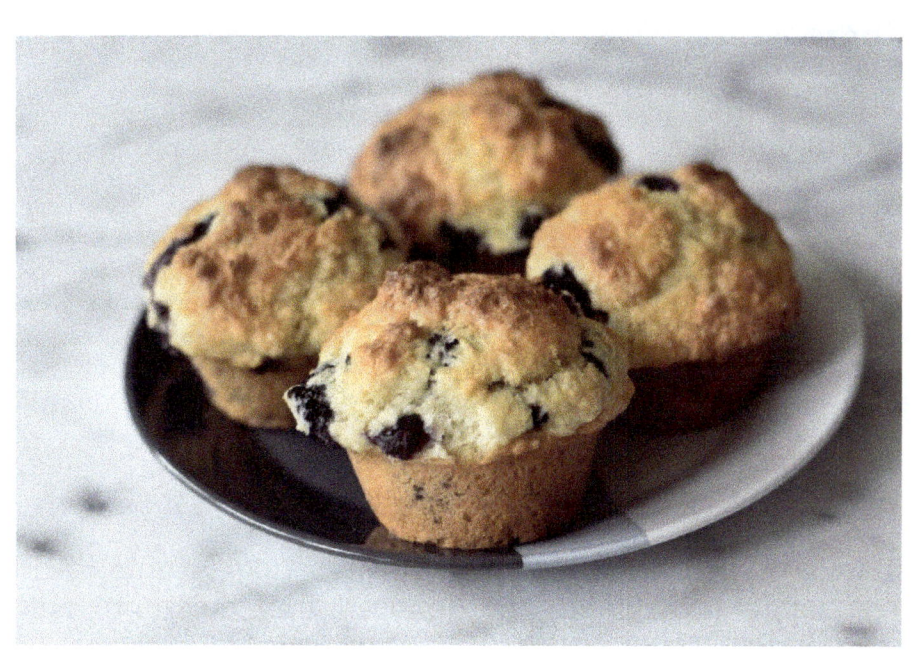

Choco Butter Brownie

Preparation Time:

10 minutes

Cooking Time:

20 minutes

Serve: 12

Ingredients:

2 eggs

1/2 tsp baking soda

2 tbsp unsweetened cocoa powder

1/4 cup Swerve

1/2 cup almond flour

1/2 cup peanut butter

2 tsp vanilla

1/3 cup coconut oil, melted

Directions:

1. In a bowl, mix together all dry ingredients. Add remaining ingredients to the bowl and mix until well combined.

2. Pour batter into the greased 8*8-inch baking dish. Select Bake mode. Set time to 20 minutes and temperature 350 F then press START.

3. The air fryer display will prompt you to ADD FOOD once the temperature is reached then place the baking dish in the air fryer basket. Serve and enjoy.

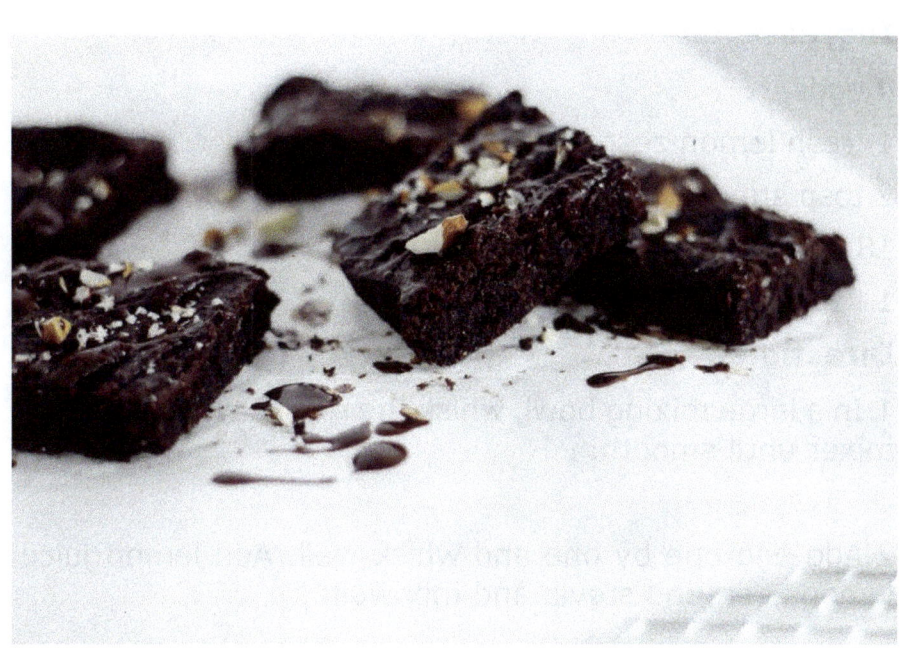

Ricotta Cake

Preparation Time:

10 minutes

Cooking Time:

55 minutes

Serve: 8

Ingredients:

4 eggs

1 fresh lemon zest

2 tbsp stevia

18 oz ricotta

1 fresh lemon juice

Directions:

1. In a large mixing bowl, whisk the ricotta with an electric mixer until smooth.

2. Add egg one by one and whisk well. Add lemon juice, lemon zest, and stevia and mix well.

3. Transfer mixture into the greased baking dish. Select Bake mode. Set time to 55 minutes and temperature 350 F then press START.

4. The air fryer display will prompt you to ADD FOOD once the temperature is reached then place the baking dish in the air fryer basket. Place cake in the refrigerator for 1-2 hours. Slice and serve

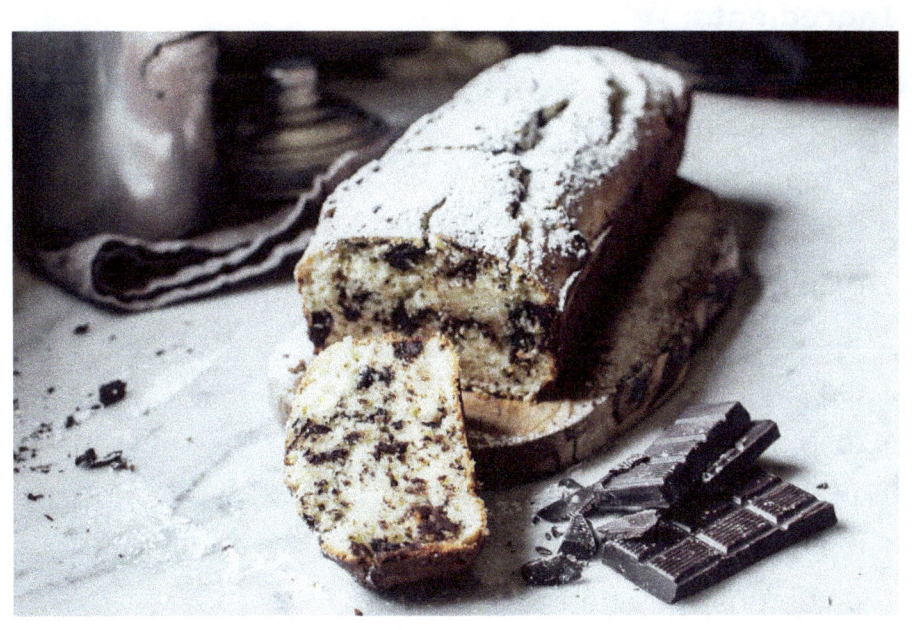

Cinnamon Nut Muffins

Preparation Time:

10 minutes

Cooking Time:

15 minutes

Serve: 12

Ingredients:

4 eggs

1/4 cup walnuts, chopped

1/2 tsp ground cinnamon

2 tsp allspice

2 tbsp butter, melted

1/2 cup Swerve

1 tsp psyllium husk

1 tbsp baking powder

1 1/2 cups almond flour

1 tsp vanilla

1/4 cup unsweetened almond milk

1/4 cup pecans, chopped

Directions:

1. Beat eggs, almond milk, vanilla, sweetener, and butter in a mixing bowl using a hand mixer until smooth.

2. Add remaining ingredients and mix until well combined. Pour batter into silicone muffin molds.

3.Select Bake mode. Set time to 15 minutes and temperature 400 F then press START.

4.The air fryer display will prompt you to ADD FOOD once the temperature is reached then place muffin molds in the air fryer basket. Serve and enjoy.

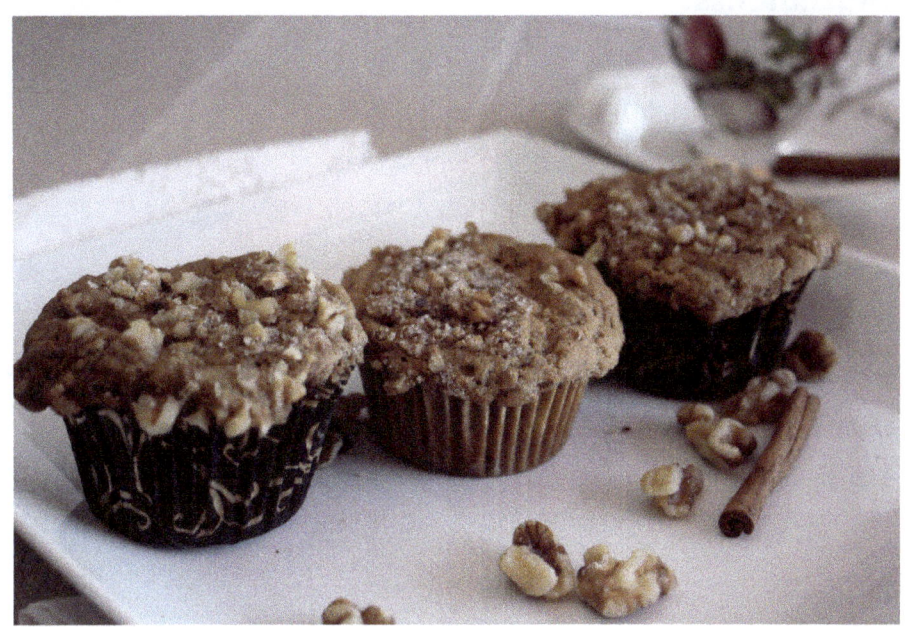

Chocolate Cheese Brownies

Preparation Time:

10 minutes

Cooking Time:

20 minutes

Serve: 12

Ingredients:

6 eggs

1/2 tsp baking powder

2/3 cup unsweetened cocoa powder

1 1/2 sticks butter, melted

4 tbsp Erythritol

4 oz cream cheese, softened

2 tsp vanilla

Directions:

1. Add all ingredients into the mixing bowl and beat until smooth. Pour mixture into the greased square baking dish.

2. Select Bake mode. Set time to 20 minutes and temperature 350 F then press START.

3. The air fryer display will prompt you to ADD FOOD once the temperature is reached then place the baking dish in the air fryer basket. Slice and serve.

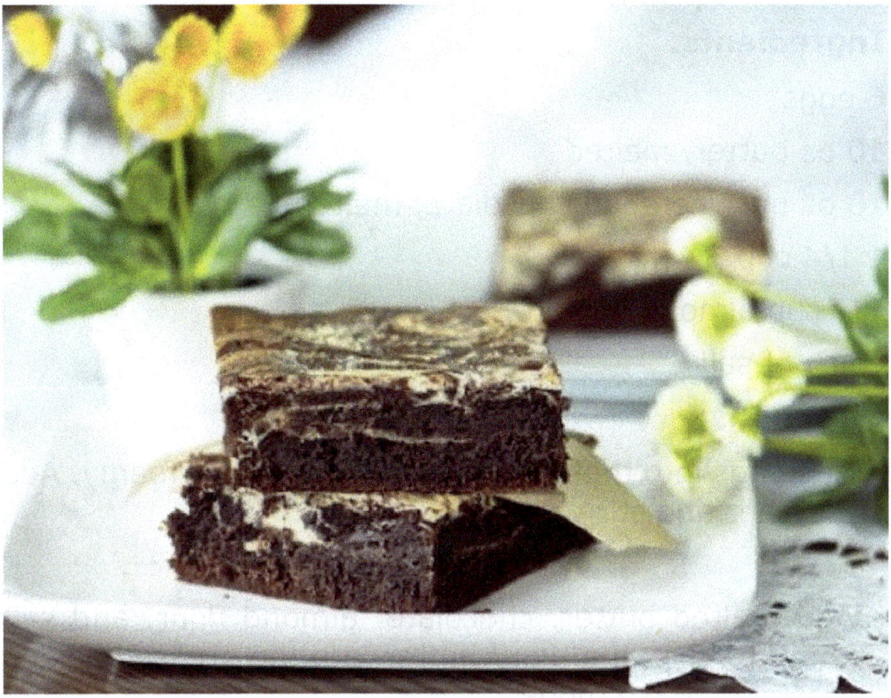

Easy Chocolate Cake

Preparation Time:

10 minutes

Cooking Time:

30 minutes

Serve: 12

Ingredients:

6 eggs

10 oz butter, melted

10 oz unsweetened chocolate, melted

1 1/4 cup Swerve

1/2 cup almond flour

Pinch of salt

Directions:

1. Add eggs into the large bowl and beat until foamy. Add sweetener and stir well.

2. Add melted butter, chocolate, almond flour, and salt and stir to combine. Pour batter into the greased baking dish. Select Bake mode.

3. Set time to 30 minutes and temperature 350 F then press START.

4. The air fryer display will prompt you to ADD FOOD once the temperature is reached then place the baking dish in the air fryer basket. Slice and serve.

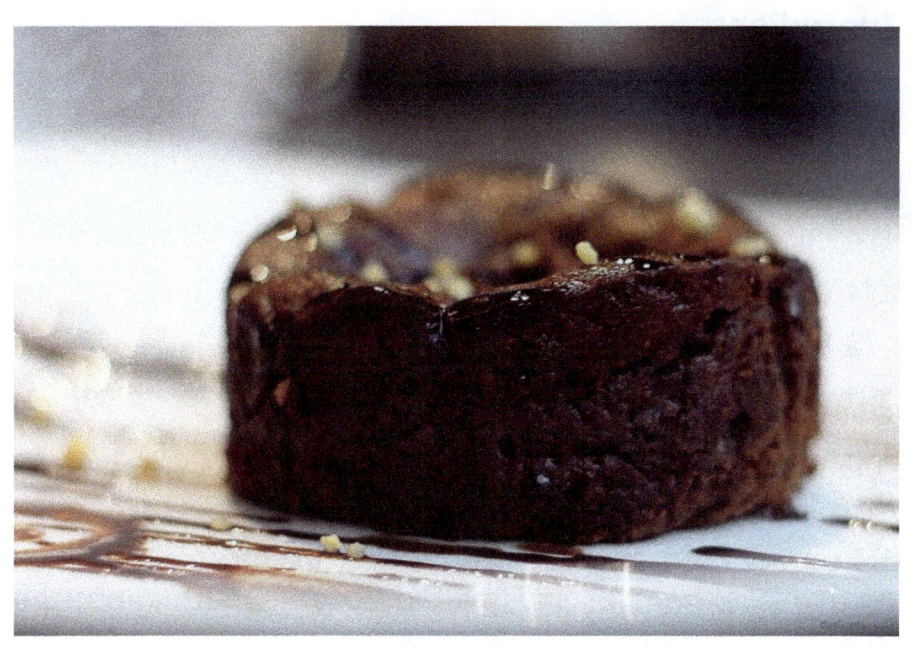

Choco Protein Brownie

Preparation Time:

10 minutes

Cooking Time:

15 minutes

Serve: 8

Ingredients:

4 egg whites

2 scoops chocolate protein powder

3 tbsp unsweetened cocoa powder

1/4 cup Erythritol

1/4 cup almond flour

1/2 tsp vanilla

3 tbsp coconut butter, melted

1/4 tsp salt

Directions:

1. In a medium bowl, mix together dry ingredients. Add egg whites, vanilla, and melted coconut butter into the mixing bowl and beat until smooth.

2. Add dry mixture into the egg white mixture and mix until well combined. Pour batter into the greased baking dish.

3. Select Bake mode. Set time to 15 minutes and temperature 300 F then press START.

4. The air fryer display will prompt you to ADD FOOD once the temperature is reached then place the baking dish in the air fryer basket. Slice and serve

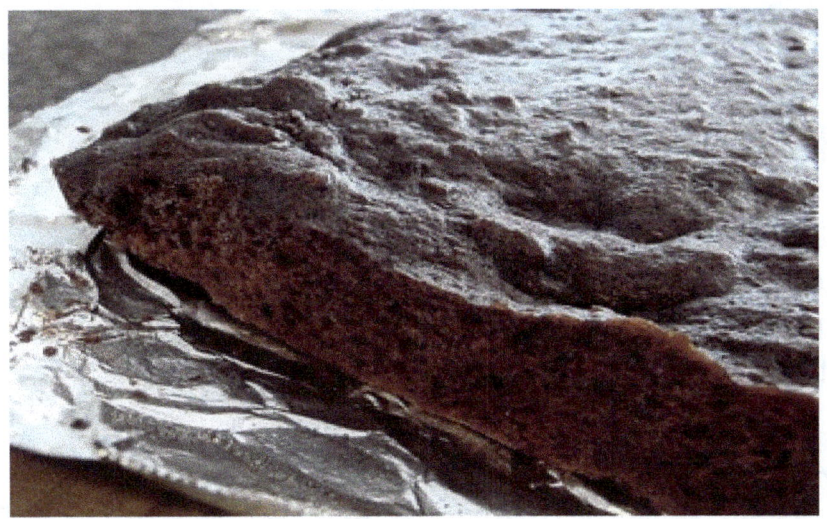

Sliced Apples

Preparation Time:

10 minutes

Cooking Time:

10 minutes

Serve: 6

Ingredients:

4 small apples, sliced

1/2 cup Swerve

2 tbsp coconut oil, melted

1 tsp apple pie spice

Directions:

1. Add apple slices in a bowl and sprinkle sweetener, apple pie spice, and coconut oil over apple and toss to coat.

2. Transfer apple slices in the baking dish. Select Air Fry mode. Set time to 10 minutes and temperature 350 F then press START.

3. The air fryer display will prompt you to ADD FOOD once the temperature is reached then place the baking dish in the air fryer basket. Serve and enjoy.

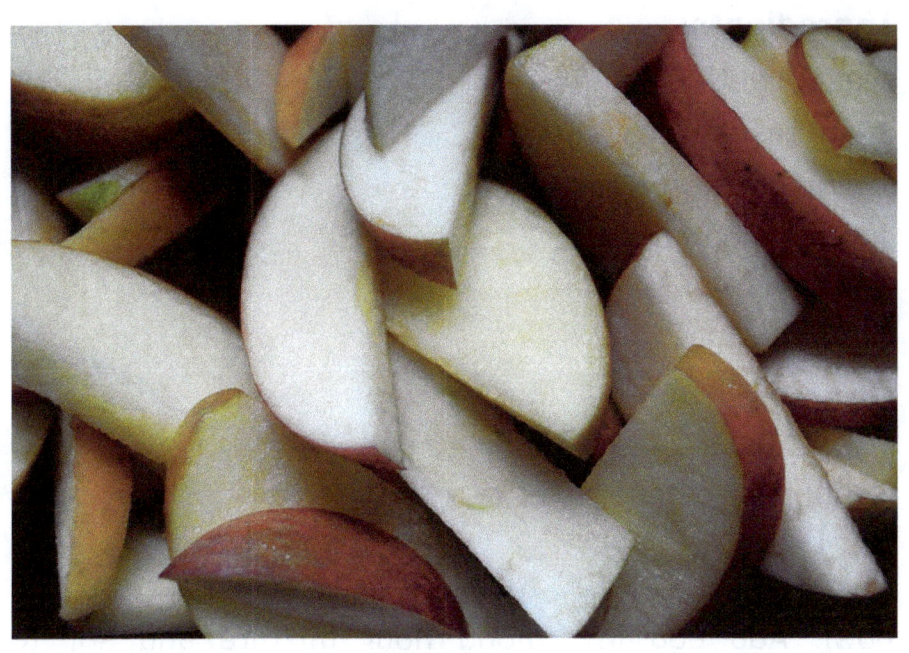

Raspberry Cobbler

Preparation Time:

10 minutes

Cooking Time:

10 minutes

Serve: 6

Ingredients:

1 egg, lightly beaten

1 cup raspberries, sliced

1 tbsp butter, melted

1 cup almond flour

2 tsp swerve

1/2 tsp vanilla

Directions:

1. Add sliced raspberries into the air fryer baking dish. Sprinkle sweetener over berries.

2. Mix together almond flour, vanilla, and butter in the bowl. Add egg in almond flour mixture and stir to combine.

3. Spread almond flour mixture over sliced berries. Cover dish with foil.

4. Select Bake mode. Set time to 10 minutes and temperature 350 F then press START.

5.The air fryer display will prompt you to ADD FOOD once the temperature is reached then place the baking dish in the air fryer basket. Serve and enjoy.

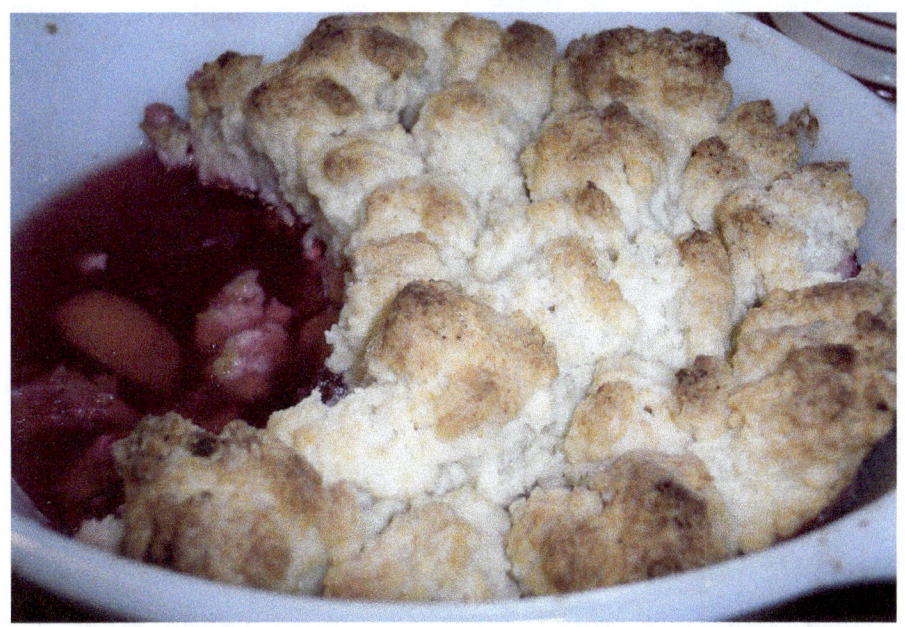

Protein Donut Balls

Preparation Time:

10 minutes

Cooking Time:

6 minutes

Serve: 16

Ingredients:

3 eggs

2 tbsp coconut oil

1/2 tsp lemon zest, grated

1 1/2 tsp apple pie spice

1 tsp baking powder

1 tbsp coconut flour

3 scoops vanilla protein powder

Directions:

1. In a large bowl, mix together protein powder, apple pie spice, baking powder, and coconut flour.

2. Add lemon zest, eggs, and coconut oil and mix until kneadable dough is forms. Place the dough onto a clean surface and knead for 10 seconds.

3. Divide dough into the sixteen pieces and roll into balls. Place the cooking tray in the air fryer basket. Place piece of parchment paper into the air fryer basket.

4. Select Air Fry mode. Set time to 6 minutes and temperature 350 F then press START.

5. The air fryer display will prompt you to ADD FOOD once the temperature is reached then place dough balls onto the parchment paper in the air fryer basket. Serve and enjoy.

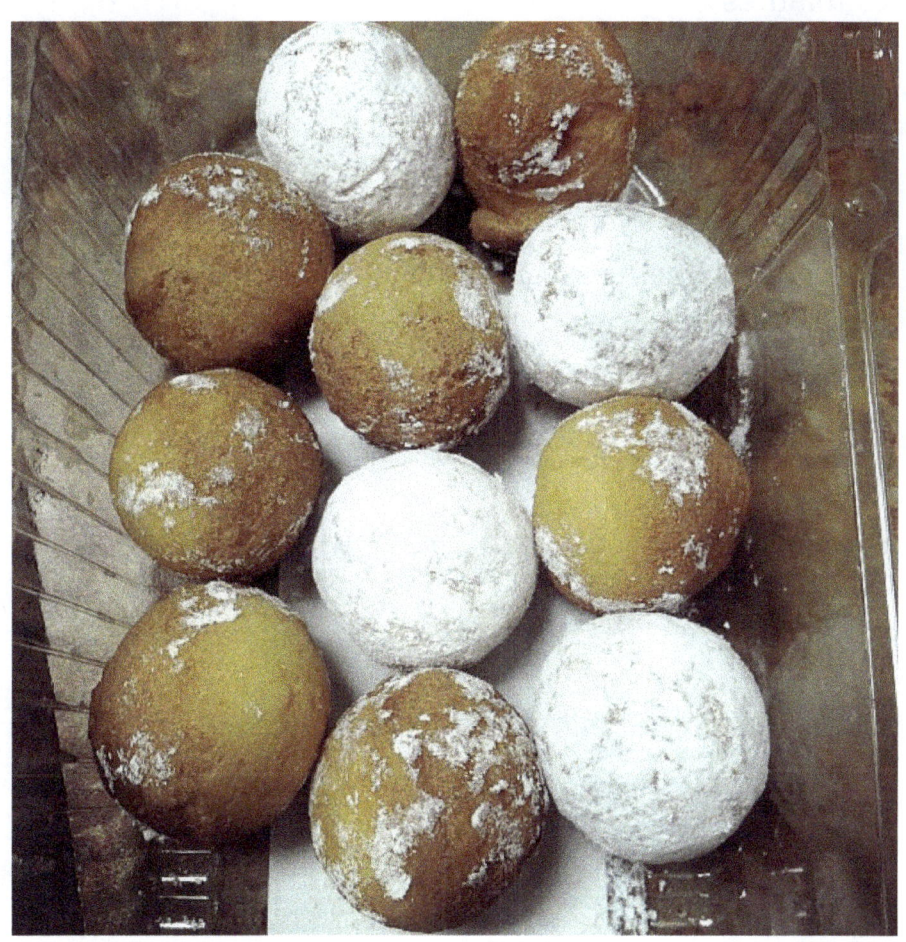

Delicious Brownie Cupcake

Preparation Time:

10 minutes

Cooking Time:

15 minutes

Serve: 6

Ingredients:

3 eggs

1/3 cup butter, melted

1/3 cup unsweetened cocoa powder

1/2 cup erythritol

1 cup almond flour

1 tbsp gelatin

Directions:

1. Add all ingredients into the bowl and stir until just combined. Pour batter into the silicone muffin molds. Select Bake mode.

2. Set time to 15 minutes and temperature 350 F then press START.

3. The air fryer display will prompt you to ADD FOOD once the temperature is reached then place muffin molds in the air fryer basket. Serve and enjoy.

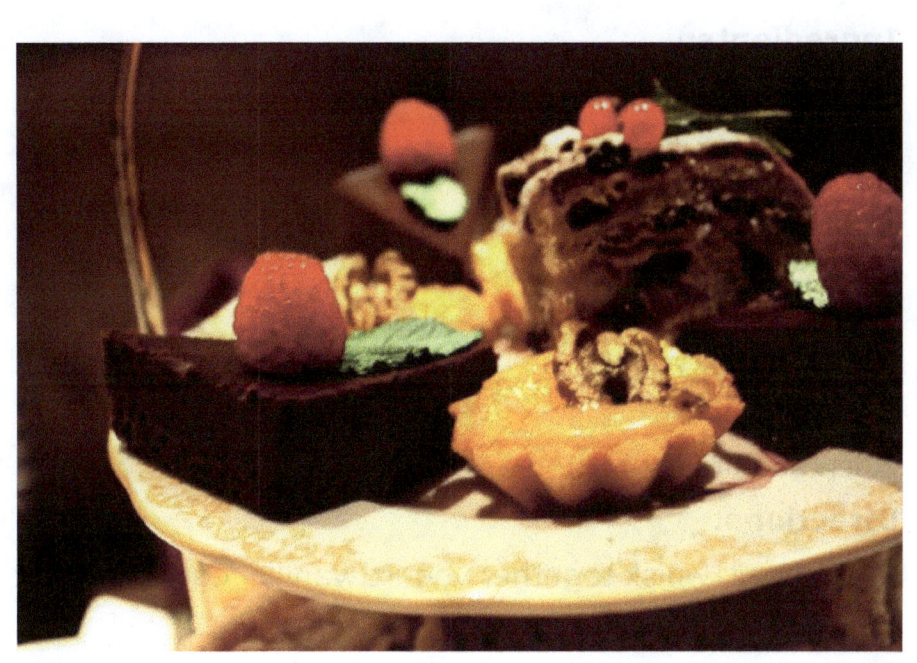

Blueberry Almond Muffins

Preparation Time:

10 minutes

Cooking Time:

30 minutes

Serve: 12

Ingredients:

3 eggs

1/2 cup fresh blueberries

2 tsp baking powder

1/4 cup Erythritol

2 1/2 cups almond flour

5.5 oz Greek yogurt

1/2 tsp vanilla

Pinch of salt

Directions:

1. In a bowl, whisk together yogurt, vanilla, eggs, and salt until smooth.

2. Add almond flour, baking powder, and sweetener and blend again until smooth.

3. Add blueberries and stir well. Pour batter into the silicone muffin molds. Select Bake mode. Set time to 30 minutes and temperature 325 F then press START.

4. The air fryer display will prompt you to ADD FOOD once the temperature is reached then place muffin molds in the air fryer basket. Serve and enjoy.

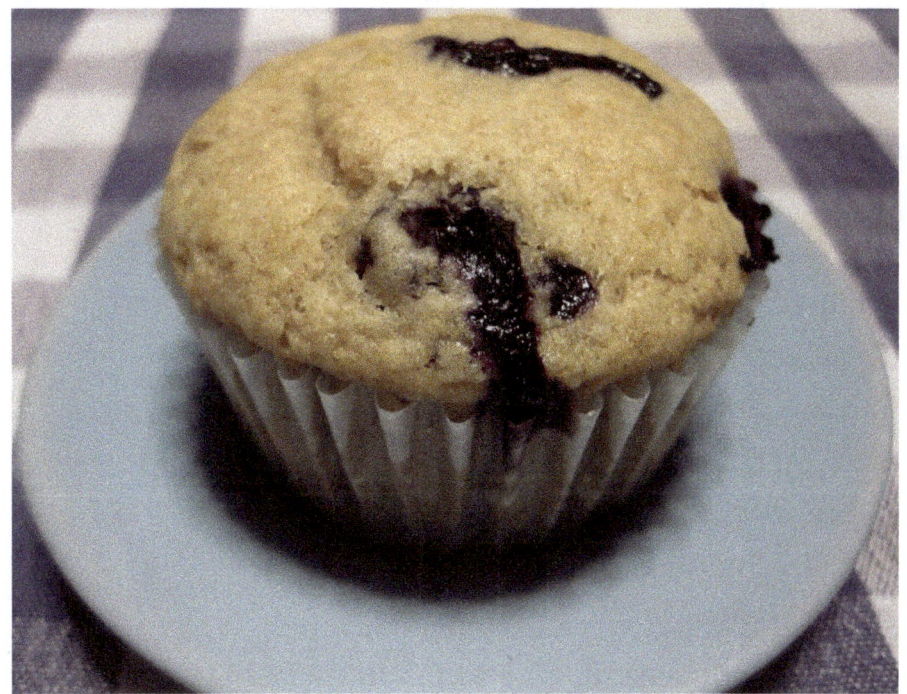

Almond Lemon Bars

Preparation Time:

10 minutes

Cooking Time:

40 minutes

Serve: 8

Ingredients:

4 eggs

1/3 cup Swerve

1 lemon zest

1/4 cup fresh lemon juice

1/2 cup butter softened

1/2 cup sour cream

2 tsp baking powder

2 cups almond flour

Directions:

1. In a bowl, beat eggs until frothy. Add butter and sour cream and beat until well combined.

2. Add sweetener, lemon zest, and lemon juice and blend well. Add baking powder and almond flour and stir until well combined.

3. Pour batter into the parchment-lined baking dish. Select Bake mode. Set time to 40 minutes and temperature 350 F then press START.

4. The air fryer display will prompt you to ADD FOOD once the temperature is reached then place the baking dish in the air fryer basket. Slice and serve.

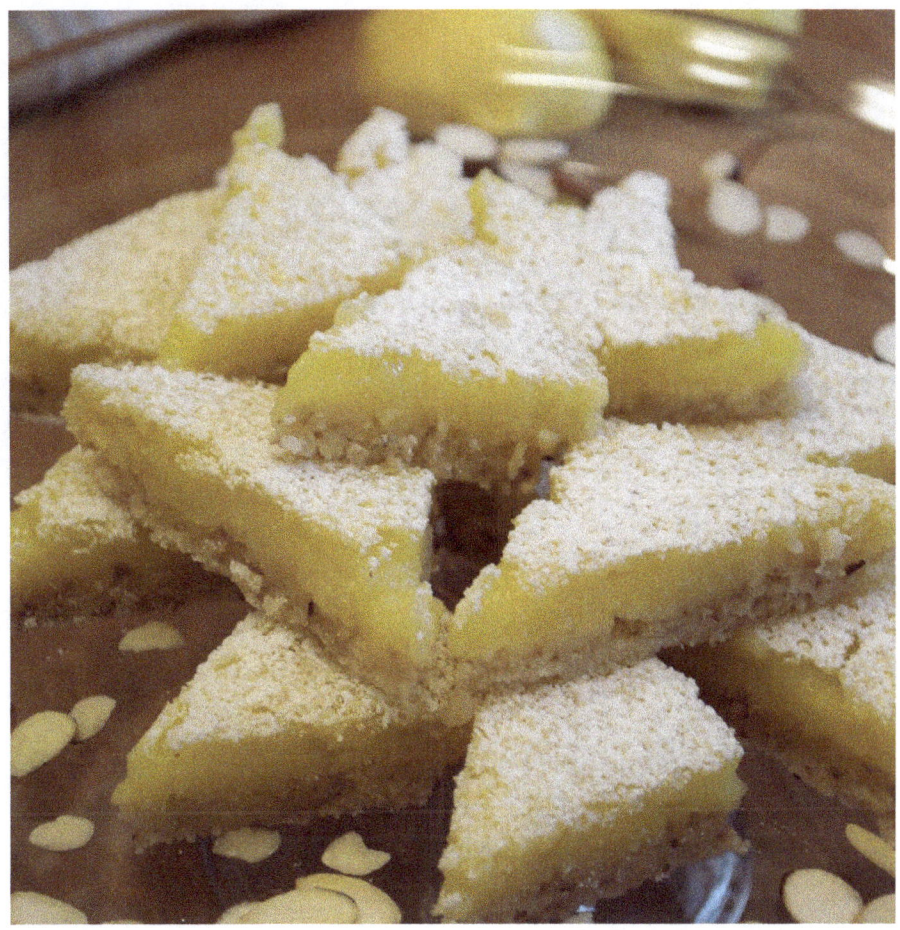

Coconut Pumpkin Custard

Preparation Time:

10 minutes

Cooking Time:

40 minutes

Serve: 6

Ingredients:

4 egg yolks

1/2 tsp cinnamon

1 tsp liquid stevia

15 oz pumpkin puree

3/4 cup coconut cream

1/8 tsp cloves

1/8 tsp ginger

Directions:

1. In a large bowl, mix pumpkin puree, cloves, ginger, cinnamon, and sweetener.

2. Add egg yolks and beat until well combined. Add coconut cream and stir well. Pour mixture into the six ramekins. Select Bake mode.

3. Set time to 40 minutes and temperature 350 F then press START.

4. The air fryer display will prompt you to ADD FOOD once the temperature is reached then place ramekins in the air fryer basket. Allow cooling completely then place in the refrigerator. Serve and enjoy.

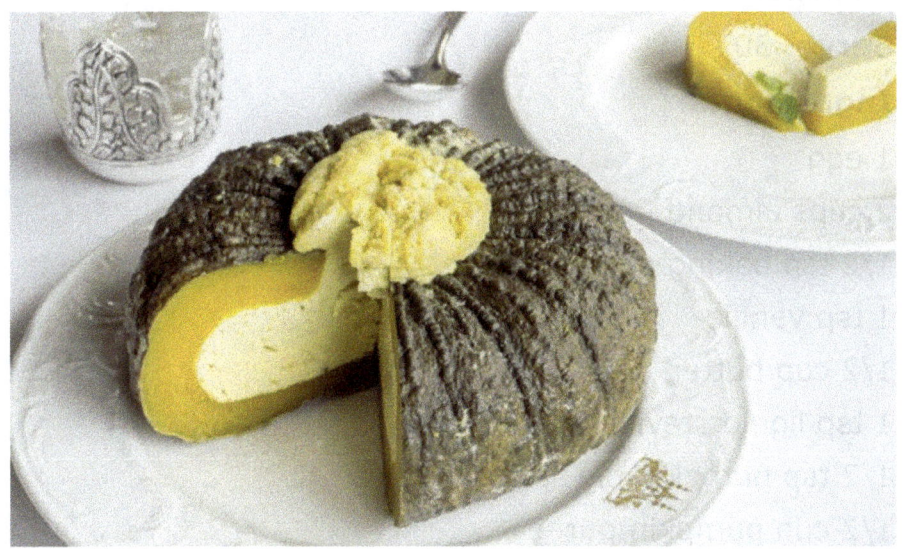

Pumpkin Cookies

Preparation Time:

10 minutes

Cooking Time:

25 minutes

Serve: 30

Ingredients:

1 egg

2 cups almond flour

1/2 tsp baking powder

1 tsp vanilla

1/2 cup butter

1 tsp liquid stevia

1/2 tsp pumpkin pie spice

1/2 cup pumpkin puree

Directions:

1. In a large bowl, add all ingredients and mix until well combined.

2. Make cookies from the mixture. Place the cooking tray in the air fryer basket. Line air fryer basket with parchment paper.

3. Select Bake mode. Set time to 25 minutes and temperature 300 F then press START.

4.The air fryer display will prompt you to ADD FOOD once the temperature is reached then place some cookies onto the parchment paper in the air fryer basket. Bake cookies in batches. Serve and enjoy.

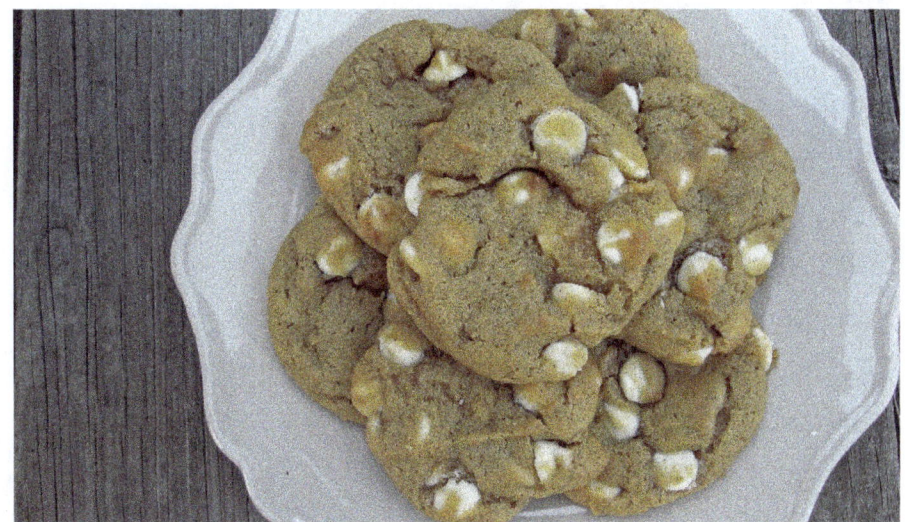

Vanilla Coconut Cake

Preparation Time:

10 minutes

Cooking Time:

20 minutes

Serve: 8

Ingredients:

5 eggs, separated

1/2 cup Swerve

1/4 cup unsweetened coconut milk

1/2 cup coconut flour

1/2 tsp baking powder

1/2 tsp vanilla

1/2 cup butter softened

Pinch of salt

Directions:

1. In a bowl, beat sweetener and butter until combined. Add egg yolks, coconut milk, and vanilla and mix well.

2. Add baking powder, coconut flour, and salt and stir well. In a separate bowl, beat egg whites until stiff peak forms. Slowly fold egg whites into the cake mixture.

3. Pour batter into the greased baking dish. Select Bake mode. Set time to 20 minutes and temperature 400 F then press START.

4.The air fryer display will prompt you to ADD FOOD once the temperature is reached then place the baking dish in the air fryer basket. Slice and serve.

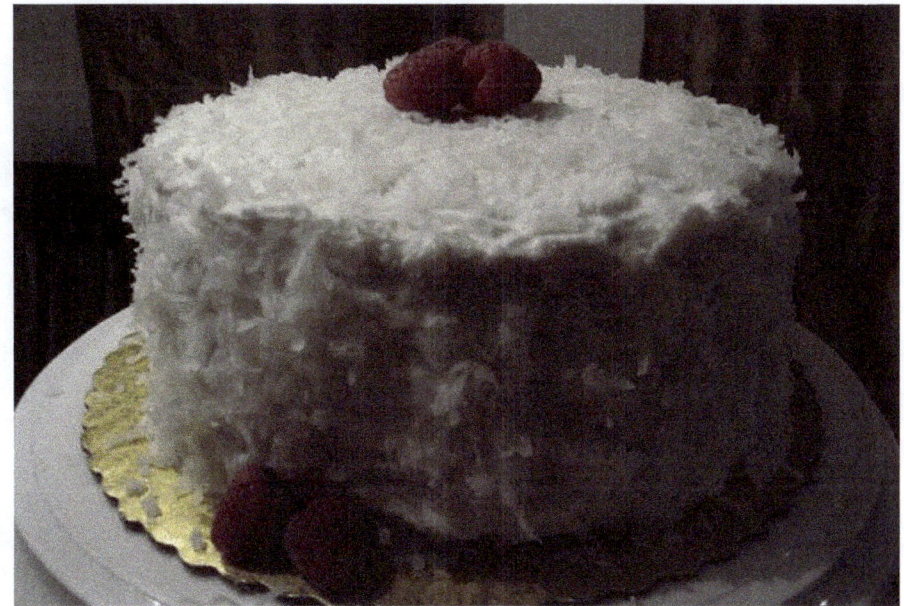

Butter Cake

Preparation Time:

10 minutes

Cooking Time:

35 minutes

Serve: 8

Ingredients:

5 eggs

6.5 oz almond flour

1/2 cup butter, softened

4 oz cream cheese, softened

1 tsp baking powder

1 tsp vanilla extract

1 cup Erythritol

Directions:

1. Add all ingredients into the mixing bowl and whisk until batter is smooth. Pour batter into the greased 9-inch baking dish.

2. Select Bake mode. Set time to 35 minutes and temperature 350 F then press START.

3. The air fryer display will prompt you to ADD FOOD once the temperature is reached then place the baking dish in the air fryer basket. Slices and serve.

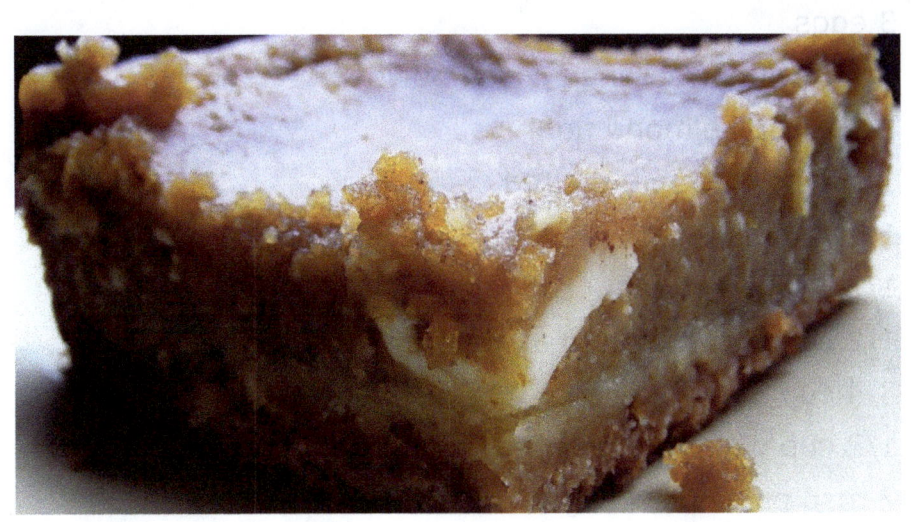

Chocolate Brownies

Preparation Time:

10 minutes

Cooking Time:

40 minutes

Serve: 12

Ingredients:

3 eggs

3/4 cup unsweetened cocoa powder

1 1/4 cups almond flour

1 cup coconut oil, melted

1 tsp vanilla

1/2 tsp vinegar

1/2 cup unsweetened almond milk

3/4 cup Swerve

1/2 cup walnuts, chopped

2 tbsp proteins collagen

1/4 tsp baking soda

Pinch of salt

Directions:

1. Add eggs, vanilla, vinegar, milk, and swerve into the large bowl and blend with a hand mixer for 2-3 minutes.

2. In a separate bowl, whisk together coconut oil, protein collagen, baking soda, cocoa powder, almond flour, and salt until combined.

3. Add egg mixture and stir until well combined. Add walnuts and fold well. Pour batter into the greased 8*8-inch baking dish.

4. Select Bake mode. Set time to 40 minutes and temperature 350 F then press START.

5. The air fryer display will prompt you to ADD FOOD once the temperature is reached then place the baking dish in the air fryer basket. Slice and serve.

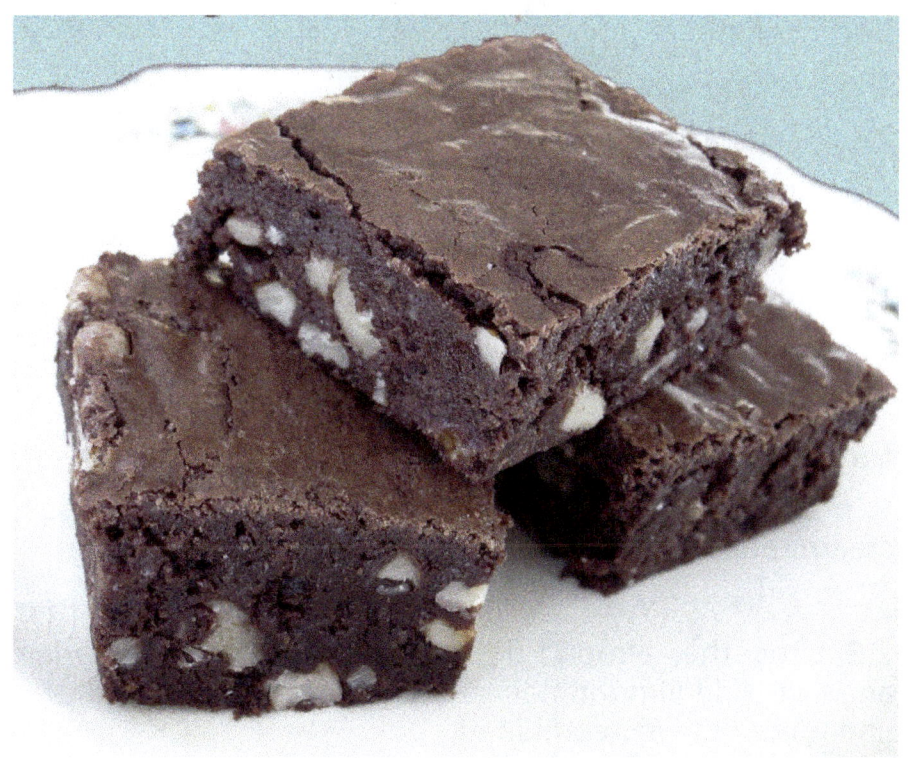

Cinnamon Strawberry Muffins

Preparation Time:

10 minutes

Cooking Time:

20 minutes

Serve: 12

Ingredients:

3 eggs

2/3 cup strawberries, diced

1 tsp cinnamon

2 tsp baking powder

2 1/2 cups almond flour

1/3 cup heavy cream

1 tsp vanilla

1/2 cup Swerve

5 tbsp butter, melted

1/4 tsp Himalayan salt

Directions:

1. In a bowl, beat together butter and swerve. Add eggs, cream, and vanilla and beat until frothy.

2. Sift together almond flour, cinnamon, baking powder, and salt. Add almond flour mixture to the wet ingredients and mix until well combined.

3. Add strawberries and fold well. Pour batter into the silicone muffin molds.

4.Select Bake mode. Set time to 20 minutes and temperature 350 F then press START.

5.The air fryer display will prompt you to ADD FOOD once the temperature is reached then place muffin molds in the air fryer basket. Serve and enjoy.

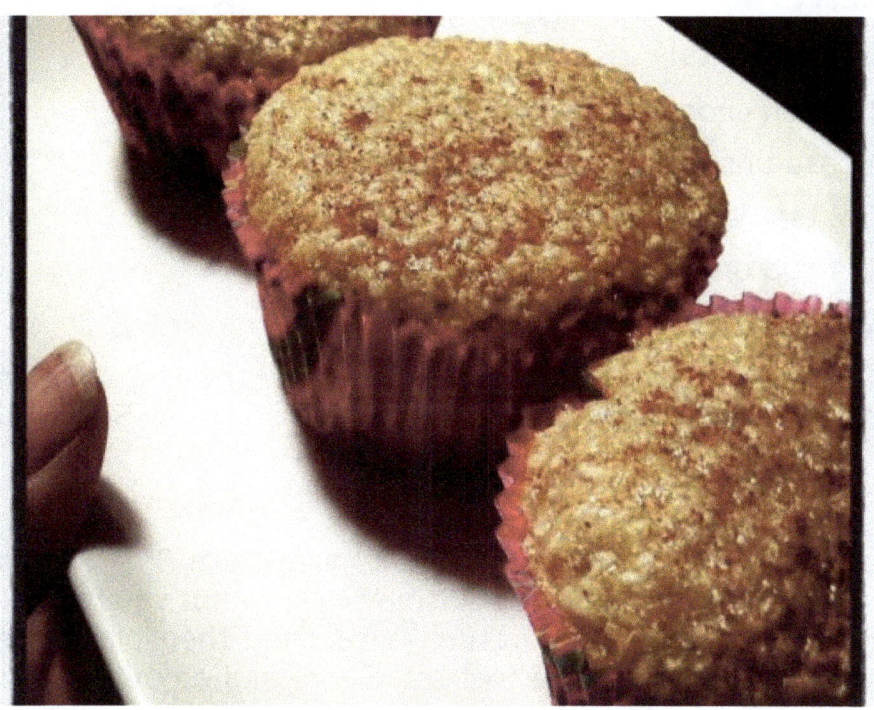

Quick Brownie

Preparation Time:

10 minutes

Cooking Time:

10 minutes

Serve: 1

Ingredients:

1 scoop chocolate protein powder

1 tbsp unsweetened cocoa powder

1/2 tsp baking powder

1/4 cup unsweetened almond milk

Directions:

1. In a ramekin mix together baking powder, protein powder, and cocoa powder. Add milk stir well. Select Ai Fry mode.

2. Set time to 10 minutes and temperature 390 F then press START. The air fryer display will prompt you to ADD FOOD once the temperature is reached then place the ramekin in the air fryer basket. Serve and enjoy.

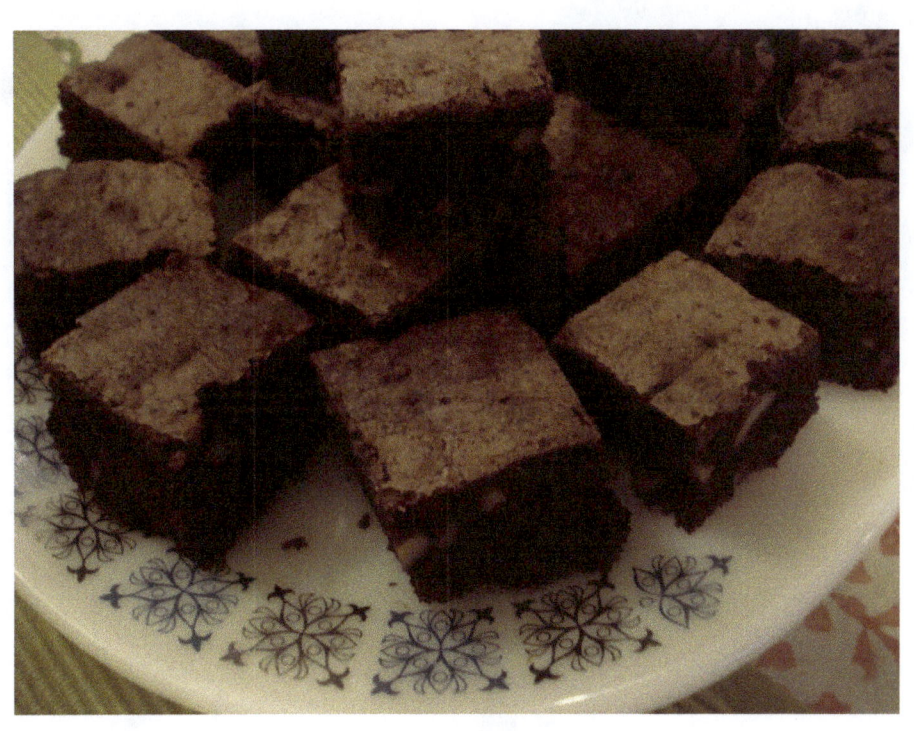

www.ingramcontent.com/pod-product-compliance
Lightning Source LLC
Chambersburg PA
CBHW070732030426
42336CB00013B/1950